KNOW

the benefits of the nutrient that can reverse or prevent arthritis

KNOW

the "wonder foods" that can back your body with energy and healthful wellbeing

KNOW

the danger signals of mineral and vitamin deficiency

KNOW

the best sources of each essential food element

You can know all these vital facts—and much, much more fascinating, healthsaving information—with

KNOW YOUR NUTRITION

the classic on good health through natural living, newly revised and updated with the latest health and nutrition developments.

KNOW YOUR NUTRITION

Linda Clark

Keats Publishing, Inc. New Canaan, Connecticut

AUTHOR'S NOTE

Due to an increasing number of letters and requests for information I can no longer answer personal letters. I am not legally allowed to prescribe, recommend or advise on individual problems. I can, however, report on research which is available in my books, articles, scientific journals and elsewhere.

KNOW YOUR NUTRITION

Pivot Health Edition published 1984
by Keats Publishing, Inc.
Copyright © 1973 by Linda Clark
Revised edition Copyright © 1981 by Linda Clark

Parts of this book were published previously in *Let's Live* magazine

ISBN: 0-87983-401-3
Library of Congress Catalog Number: 80-84437

Printed in the United States of America

Keats Publishing, Inc.
27 Pine Street (Box 876)
New Canaan, Connecticut 06840

Contents

In reference lists:

Ibid. is used to refer to the work in the note immediately preceding.

op. cit., with author's name, stands in place of the title of a work cited earlier in each chapter list.

1
Should You Take Vitamins and Minerals?

Nutrition is a young and growing science. Probably one of the greatest controversies of this century is concerned with the question of whether or not we should take vitamins and minerals. More and more people *are* taking them in spite of the fact that the government agency, the Food and Drug Administration (FDA), looks upon them with disfavor, particularly if used in substantial amounts. The FDA claims that vitamin and mineral supplements are not necessary for health because our food contains everything we need for health.

Many authorities challenge this statement and supply sobering proof to the contrary, as you will see. The FDA also believes that only faddists consider chemical fertilizers and insecticides poisonous for the land upon which our food is grown. They do not believe that soil depletion (from continuous overcropping) can result in deficient foods and consequently in malnourished people who eat these foods. The FDA also refuses to admit that the processing of the foods we buy in most stores can interfere with quality. And they categorically deny that much disease is due to improper diet, which now allows up to 5,000 questionable additives.

Let's face it: for the most part, we are what we eat. The type of fuel we take into our bodies is a large factor in determining our health. Vitamins and minerals should be present in our diet in some form: in our food, or as additional supplements, or both. But assimilation is also important.

Here are some questions many people are asking about this crucial health and food problem. The questions, with the answers from experts, should help clarify the confusion so that you can decide for yourself whether or not *you* wish to take vitamin and mineral supplements.

ISN'T IT TRUE THAT AMERICA IS THE BEST-FED COUNTRY IN THE WORLD?

Although our national food supply is undeniably the most *abundant* in the world, much of it is grown in depleted soils and/or processed, refined, precooked (as in convenience foods and TV dinners), frozen and stored for prolonged periods. As a result, nutrients are diminished or lost from the food supply, and the public is getting many "empty calories."

Government surveys prove the point with these statistics:

Millions of teenagers have been found to be malnourished.

Millions of adults, even those with high incomes, do not have diets adequate for maintaining health.

American men rank thirteenth in world health; American women, sixth.

As examples of inadequate nutrition, 52 million people (29 percent of the American population) are receiving inadequate calcium; and 45 million are deficient in vitamin C.

Remember, this is *government* information based on actual tests. Therefore, by taking vitamin and mineral supplements, you can provide nutritional insurance for yourself; you can provide a margin of safety to compensate for the nutrients you are not getting in your diet.

WHY DO CHEMICAL FERTILIZERS DISTURB THE SOIL AND THE PLANTS (FOOD) GROWN THERE?

Chemical fertilizers stimulate growth, but, according to Dr. John Bircher of Switzerland: "To ensure the growth of wholesome plant tissues and also for their protection against disease, cultivated plants and vegetables require a *slow* balanced feeding of nutritious substances."

Chemicals have also become responsible, as you know, for polluting the soil, air and water, as well as the birds, fish and animals. The late Dr. William A. Albrecht, soil scientist and Dean Emeritus of the Department of Soils at the University of Missouri after fifty years there, made the following statements:

"Destruction of the soil by man's increasing use of chemicals is moving the U.S. and the rest of the world toward a disastrous famine.

"Soil fertility will decrease to the point that many farmers will fail economically.

"Man has been plundering the soil to such an extent that he is destroying its fertility. As a result the protein in our grain crops [alone] is rapidly diminishing. For example, the protein content of Kansas wheat ranged from 16 to 19 percent in 1940; in 1968, it ranged only from 11 to 13 percent.

"You've got to have fertile soil to grow healthy plants. Only healthy plants can provide proper feed for animals and humans.

"If you're not nourished properly, you won't survive. That's why sickness is increasing."

In other words, in the opinion of this scientist, who spent his life studying and teaching, sick soils result in sick animals and sick people. Extensive tests supply proof.

WHY ARE FOODS PROCESSED AND WHAT IS WRONG WITH THE PRACTICE?

Alan H. Nittler, M.D., tells us: "There are at least 3,000 different chemicals allowed in our foods, one way or another, and about 8,000 different ones in our total environment that we can eat, drink, breathe or touch. These chemicals include poisons, drugs, preservatives, sweeteners, softeners, alkalizers, acidifiers, hormones, dyes, antioxidants and hydrogenators. Some are poisonous and some are not. *But all are abnormal to the human body and must be neutralized or excreted or else disease or death results.*"

Even though the government has banned some of the chemical additives because they have been proved by laboratory tests to be toxic, even cancer-causing in some cases, others have been allowed to remain in the food due to entreaties by the food processors who find their use profitable.

In addition to being processed, much of our food is refined. Important nutrients are removed from natural foods to prevent spoilage and assure a longer shelf life, thus eliminating financial loss for manufacturer and grocer alike. Refining food causes:

Loss of vitamins B and E in the milling of grains

Loss of essential fatty acids

Complete loss of vitamins and minerals in the manufacturing of white sugar, and some loss in the manufacturing of "raw" sugar

Loss of vitamin C in precooking (of convenience foods), storing and prolonged freezing

For those who contend that even if nutrients are removed from grains for breads and cereals, these foods are at least "enriched," usually eight or more natural vitamins and minerals are removed and only three synthetic ones are substituted. What is the effect of these enriched grain products on health? Roger J. Williams, Ph.D., director of the Clayton Biochemical Foundation at the University of Texas, found that commercially enriched bread is so low in nutrients that of sixty-four laboratory rats fed nothing but enriched bread, forty died of malnutrition and the growth of the survivors was severely stunted.

Because natural nutrients are so fragile and spoil so easily, some wit has said quite correctly: "Eat only the foods that spoil, but eat them before they do." Fortunately, many unprocessed natural foods are available at most health stores.

For self-protection we should raise our own food if possible.

WHAT ARE ORGANIC FOODS?
WHERE CAN I FIND THEM?

The word "organic" is being challenged in high places. Organic foods are those grown on properly nourished soil and not exposed to chemical fertilizers, pesticides, sprays or other pollutants. Due to the increasing demand, organic foods are becoming more readily available from some farmers, health stores and other food outlets. However, insist on proof on the label that the organic foods you buy are free of pollutants. Because organic foods take longer to grow and require more effort by the farmer than mass-production through chemicals and pesticides, they will probably be more expensive, if you can find them at all. Many of them must be shipped thousands of miles, since so few local sources are available. However, in terms of health, they are a good value. One expert says: "Our food and, in turn, ourselves suffer from nutritional imbalances."

Four doctors, quoted in Ehrenfried Pfeiffer's book, *Biodynamic Farming and Gardening* (a form of organic farming and gardening by natural methods), state that their patients were healthier as a result of eating whole, organic foods.

So search everywhere for organic foods (or raise your own). Look for organic farmers in your own neighborhood. Write *Organic Gardening and Farming,* Customer's Service, Emmaus, Pennsylvania 18049, and/or Natural Foods Associates, Atlanta, Texas 75551. And insist upon *real* organic produce. One spokesman for the Dietetics Food Industry, warns that all that glitters may not be gold. He recommends that organic food must *really* be organic, be stamped with the producer's name and guarantee, and not be a substitute to be palmed off to the unsuspecting public just to make a fast buck.

WHAT ARE VITAMINS?

There is a definition of a vitamin in the 1939 Handbook of the Department of Agriculture. This volume is called *Food and Life,* and is one of the masterpieces of nutritional knowledge, far ahead of its time. The definition states that "vitamins are substances that are essential for life and growth." (This definition applies also to minerals.)

Another definition of a vitamin is given by Rebecca Kirby, in reporting nutritional research for Natural Food Associates, an organization long headed by Joe D. Nichols, M.D. She says: "The foods one eats (or should eat) are the primary source of the life-supporting nutrients."

WHAT ABOUT THOSE UNIVERSITY NUTRITIONISTS WHO SAY WE DON'T NEED TO TAKE SUPPLEMENTS, JUST EAT A GOOD DIET?

Such statements as these mystified me, too, until I learned what was going on. In most cases the answer seems to be that the huge vested interests—including the food processors, some drug companies, and even the American Medical Association (AMA) and the FDA—perhaps began to realize that nutritional foods and supplements, plus natural, unprocessed foods, were becoming a threat to their financial survival.

More than once a campaign against such foods and supplements has been attempted, and key spokesmen were asked to attack health foods and supplements. There is written proof that some universities were subsidized by these vested interests in return for the attacks against natural foods and supplements by members of their faculty.[1] Some doctors and members of universities, however, may be entirely innocent of collaboration. A growing number are becoming concerned, even alarmed, over the problem.

WHAT DOES RDA MEAN?

RDA stands for *Recommended Dietary Allowances* which apply to the so-called needs of vitamin and mineral potencies for people of different ages, sex, etc. These RDAs, issued every four years, are generally held in contempt by many professional nutritionists, nutritionally oriented doctors and manufacturers of nutritional supplements, because they are so low.

Many of these detractors believe that the RDA levels are dominated by the food industry. They point out that the nutrients are determined on the basis of animal, not human studies, and are behind the times in knowledge. Dr. Charles T. McGee, M.D. in his book *How to Survive Modern Technology* (Keats Publishing) states: "The RDA values have become the backbone of the analytic approach to nutrition . . . [yet] current RDA levels are set at values which will [only] sustain life. There is much evidence that higher levels . . . would help millions of people prevent degenerative diseases . . . Dr. Linus Pauling has stated that rather than keeping us in good health the current levels of the RDAs . . . will keep us in a state of poor health."

Manufacturers are required by the FDA to list these RDAs on labels of supplements, or else run the risk of not having their products be accepted for sale to the public.

What many people do not know is that there are *two* sets of RDAs, each set controlled by a different organization. The original RDAs are selected by the Food and Nutrition Board of the National Academy of Sciences, which honestly admits that their RDAs are based on available nutritional knowledge of "practically all healthy persons." (Their goal, they claim, is to maintain health, not treat disease.) They state, "We are well aware that present knowledge of nutritional needs is incomplete."

On the other hand, the group which insists on RDAs appearing on labels is the Food and Drug Administration (FDA) which apparently "borrows" the RDAs as researched and issued by the National Academy of Sciences (NAS). (The FDA is said to use the highest level of the male allowance of the NAS, an allowance which is to the FDA's credit.) Even so, the NAS warns the public, "Recommended Dietary Allowances (RDA) should not be confused with United States Recommended Daily Allowances (USRDA), a set of values derived by the Food and Drug Administration as standards for nutritional labelling." (From National Academy of Sciences: *Recommended Dietary Allowances,* Eighth edition, 1974, available for sale from NAS, 2101 Constitution Ave., Washington, D.C. 20418.)

According to research, they are a mere drop in the health bucket. Dr. Roger J. Williams says: "The building of metabolic machinery cannot possibly take place if even one little cog is missing. Adequate food must contribute the total package. A food or food mixture (or choice of supplements), *in order to support life,* must not merely supply six vitamins, five minerals and four amino acids (protein factors). It must supply the *full* quota: everything that is needed to build body machinery."

The Food and Nutrition Board believes, like the FDA, that we should get our nutrients from food. Yet a recent report states that 95 percent of our food is being tampered with. It is subject to unbelievable processing to increase sales or shelf life. Many vitamins are removed and a few synthetics, if any, are substituted.

Can you determine the precise amount of vitamins and minerals that should be present in each food you buy in order to protect your health? Robert S. Harris, Ph.D., one of our most distinguished nutritionists, a member of the Department of Nutrition and Food Science at the Massachusetts Institute of Technology (MIT), answers this question with a resounding "No!" There are too many variables in the foods, and *you* can't tell with the naked eye what is in them. But a machine can.

There is an X-ray type of machine, used by Dr. Firman E. Bear, at Rutgers University, that can see into the innards of vegetables and fruits. Although two carrots may look alike to you, to the machine the nutrients may show up as high in one carrot and practically nil in another.

Our food producers, by picking fruits green for shipping, storing them for a long time, blanching and freezing them for long periods, and precooking them as in convenience foods, are not providing you with the nutrients you think you are getting—or are paying for. All these processes cause loss of vitamin/mineral content and shortchange *you*. But that is not all.

Supermarkets know that you do know the brighter the color of a food, the higher the vitamin content. So some of them throw hidden, colored spotlights on the display of their fresh produce so that the green vegetables look greener, yellow vegetables yellower and meats redder. But put these foods in natural daylight, and you will be startled at their anemic appearance.

This is why dyes are also used for oranges in some states, sweet potatoes, red-skinned white potatoes and packaged foods. The fact that some of these dyes have been found, even by the FDA, to cause cancer, but are still allowed to remain in the food to help protect the income of the manufacturer, is never mentioned. And did you know that there is often an aroma-wafter hidden behind the bread section? It throws out tantalizing synthetic odors of freshly baked bread to entice customers to buy something that has had most of the natural vitamins and minerals removed, with a few synthetics added as replacements, and has been spiked with preservatives that have, in many cases, been proved poisonous.

This does not mean that there is nothing safe at a supermarket. Many of us have to fall back upon it for some of our supplies. But you *must* use your eyes and read labels! The listing of some chemical ingredients is required on the labels. But I have long said that if you cannot pronounce the names of the chemicals in the food, don't buy them.

It is true that because of the FDA's recommendation the nutritional contents of foods are listed on the labels by the manufacturers. But many of these labels are difficult to understand, for they are too technical or do not state the proportions of nutrients included. This brings us back full circle to the fact that in order to be *sure* we are getting our full supply of nutrients in our diet, we probably need vitamin and mineral supplements. Due to public demand, some supermarkets are beginning to sell some health foods as well as supplements.

WHY DO MOST DOCTORS CONDEMN OR FAIL TO SUGGEST VITAMIN AND MINERAL SUPPLEMENTS?

Perhaps you have already found that when you ask your doctor if you should take vitamins or minerals, he gives one of these answers: (a) they are not necessary; (b) they won't hurt you; or (c) a drug, which he would rather prescribe, will do the job better and quicker. However, drugs *suppress* symptoms instead of curing them (for example, an aspirin relieves a headache, but does not remove the cause), whereas good nutrition helps the body to rebuild itself. This takes longer than drugs, but the results are eventually more satisfactory. Some doctors use both drugs for quick relief and nutrition for body/health rebuilding.

The reason so many doctors fail to prescribe, and instead condemn, vitamin and mineral supplements (although more and more are actually prescribing them in addition to drugs) is because they were not taught nutrition in medical schools. Miles H. Robinson, M.D., who acted as cross-examiner of witnesses in FDA hearings against vitamins, minerals and health foods, reported: "It is highly significant that [even] FDA witnesses have repeatedly testified that the average doctor is woefully ignorant about vitamin deficiencies."

There appears to be another reason why some doctors prescribe drugs instead of vitamin and mineral supplements plus a highly nutritious diet. As Omar Garrison states in his book: "There is a cozy liaison which, from its inception, has existed between the FDA and the AMA and sometimes between the federal agency and large drug manufacturers or food processors."[2]

George W. Crane, Ph.D., M.D., in his foreword in

the same book, states: "In my syndicated newspaper column I have described the FDA as the political Charlie McCarthy on the knee of the American Medical Association, for it often parrots the orders from the AMA home office in Chicago with or without any convincing sufficient evidence.

"As a member of the AMA myself, I appreciate many of its worthy motives. But I don't let it do my scientific thinking for me on all matters, for it has often been proved wrong."

Another reason the AMA discourages the use of supplements is startling. In a health magazine published by the AMA for the general public, this statement appeared: "The greater danger is that people use vitamins to treat their own illnesses *instead of going to doctors.* [Emphasis mine.] This self-medication is a greater danger to the public than the danger of taking an overdose of vitamins."[3]

But what are you going to do if the doctor is not getting you well? Taking such harmless food substances as vitamins and minerals, even if self-administered, in overdoses (a rare occurrence) is far different from taking dangerous drugs even when doctor-administered.

In China, for generations the people paid doctors to keep them well. When they got sick, the payments stopped. If more doctors in other countries would use nutrition to keep their patients well, they would be more highly respected. A few have already learned this lesson and have shifted from drugs to nutritional treatment with great success. The story of how one doctor accomplished this is explained in his book, *A New Breed of Doctor.*[4] It can be done, although this doctor was severely disciplined for practicing natural nutrition: his license was revoked.

WHICH AND HOW MANY VITAMINS AND MINERALS SHOULD ONE TAKE?

This question is one basic reason for writing this book. As a contributing editor to the magazine, *Let's Live*, I am asked this question by many people. They become irate when I answer that I do not know. To begin with, even if I did know, I would not be allowed to tell them, since this would constitute prescribing without a license. But it is true that neither I nor anyone else really knows the answer. The reason: *everyone is different.*

One of the greatest experts on this subject of individual differences is Roger J. Williams, Ph.D. Dr. Williams is the discoverer of one of the B vitamins, pantothenic acid. He is also the author of several books, including two on individual differences, namely, *You Are Extraordinary*[5] and *Biochemical Individuality.*[6] In these books are pictures of some of the human organs. One page of pictures shows thirteen different stomachs, each unlike the other. A page of pictures of human hearts shows that these, too, vary in shape and size. And although anatomy teaches that certain organs are supposed to be located in certain places in the body, Dr. Williams shows proof that they are not always in the place they are supposed to be.

Since organs vary in shape and location, it will not come as a surprise to learn that they can also vary in the way they work. Nor do the glands, our body machinery, release the secretions in like manner. Some people, Dr. Williams points out, have plenty of hydrochloric acid for good digestion; others have none at all. Nutritional needs of the body also vary. One study reported by Dr. Williams showed a variation of calcium needed from person to person ranging from 222 to 1,018 milligrams (mg.) daily.

Even the need for vitamin A in rats of the same species showed all manner of variation. As for human subjects, Dr. Williams tells of a man who thrived for twenty-two months on a diet practically free of vitamin A, whereas a physician reported a woman patient who required 50,000 units a day to keep well. Dr. Williams also states that one person may need ten times as much pantothenic acid as another. So there is no rule of thumb, except our own individual differences.

DO RELIABLE EXPERTS BELIEVE IT IS ALL RIGHT TO TAKE SUPPLEMENTS?

Yes. Various scientists and nutritional physicians urge supplementation. Dr. Williams says: "It is my viewpoint that each individual has a substantial responsibility for ordering his own life, including his consumption of food. If each will take advantage of the unity of nature, diversify his food, avoid too much refined food, cultivate body wisdom and use nutritional supplements when informed judgment so dictates, I am sure that better health will be the reward."

Dr. Williams is also the author of the excellent book, *Nutrition Against Disease*,[7] which supplies scientific laboratory proof that what he calls "supernutrition" can eliminate or reduce many of mankind's serious health problems, including mental illness, cancer, birth defects, premature aging, heart disease, obesity and arthritis. He says supernutrition means that living cells thrive when furnished with an optimum environment, which consists of *at least* forty known nutrients combined in proper proportions, essential to health.

HOW DO WE KNOW WHAT CONSTITUTES TOO MANY VITAMINS FOR THE AVERAGE PERSON?

We don't. Each person is a law unto himself. Dr. Williams does not believe there is such a thing as an average person. He believes, and has proved again and again with tests on laboratory animals, that *we cannot generalize* that everyone needs precisely the same amount of vitamins and minerals. He summarizes: "We know that individual human beings have great diversity in human nutritional needs. If we accept the principles, then it follows that we must suspect the prevalence of nutritional disease in any group of people who are fed uniformly a diet designed for an average member of the group."

In other words, since no two people are alike, their nutritional needs are not alike.

WHAT IF YOU TAKE MANY VITAMINS AND MINERALS AND DO NOT GET THE DESIRED RESULTS?

There are factors that rob the body of vitamins. Check the following list to determine if one or more might be your problem.[8]

    Migraine headache (a stress)
    Gallbladder disturbance
    Colitis, gastritis
    Overactive thyroid (burns up food too fast)
    Surgical stress
    Loss of teeth, or poor-fitting dentures
    Heart disease
    Pregnancy
    Diarrhea

Lack of assimilation due to deficiencies of digestive juices (such as hydrochloric acid, bile and pepsin), poor chewing, etc.

Excessive sweating (which causes loss of water-soluble vitamins)

Hemorrhages

Burns

Severe colds

Intestinal parasites (tests show they exist in 94 out of 200 people.)

Overactive kidneys

Aging (causes poor assimilation)

Excessive physical activity

Infections

Smoking (destroys vitamin C)

Aspirin (destroys vitamin C)

Alcohol (destroys vitamin B)

Light (destroys vitamin B-2, in food overexposed to light)

Exposure to air (destroys vitamins A and C)

Excessive fluids (destroys vitamin B)

Antibiotics (upset intestinal flora and self-manufacture of B vitamins)

Antacids (destroy vitamin B and deter digestion of protein and minerals)

Stress (destroys vitamin C)

Laxatives

Chlorinated water

Polluted water

Polluted air

Drugs and sleeping pills

Rancid foods

Discarding cooking water, or cooking in too much water (leaches vitamins B and C)

Soaking foods before cooking (destroys vitamins B and C)

Adding soda to green or yellow vegetables (destroys vitamin B)

Exposure to lead, mercury, fumes from gasoline, paint and cleaning fluids, and many, many more.

HOW CAN WE HANDLE STRESS NUTRITIONALLY?

We are living in times of great stress. Air pollution, water pollution, drug pollution, food pollution and even thought pollution are coming at us from every direction. This stress, or collection of stresses, is taking its toll on our minds, emotions and bodies. In order to withstand them, we need all the help we can get.

The well-worn phrase, "A sound mind in a sound body," makes more sense than ever before. What affects one department of the body also affects the other; we cannot separate them. We can try to control our emotions, but if we have little energy, we become easily depressed and hampered in facing even the little things in life, to say nothing of the big ones. The majority of the world is suffering from lack of energy, aches and pains and is looking for help in aspirin, sleeping pills, pep pills, tranquilizers or psychedelic drugs with the blind hope that somehow these temporary measures will magically erase all their mental, emotional and physical problems. Unfortunately, it is not that easy. This is putting the cart before the horse.

It is interesting that the Hunzas and other tribes who are healthy have had no crime, in addition to having no need for doctors. They have no need for policemen, jails or other correctional or mental institutions. Their outstanding characteristic is that they are cheerful. They are never known to fight or to feel depressed. They feel *good*, are bursting with vitality and health and can cope with any problem.

This is the greatest dividend of good health: buoyancy, joie de vivre. Such health comes mainly from good nutrition, which we need as a mainstay as never before. Good nutrition is our one main hope of achieving and maintaining good health, and developing resistance to disease.

But how do we achieve good health? Again, our bodies are no better than the fuels or building materials we put into them. These building materials, or nutrients—which include vitamins, minerals and proteins—have been established by laboratory analyses as components of our body and need to be replaced regularly. They provide the energy, resistance and vitality that make your problems soluble rather than irritating and insoluble.

IS IT TRUE THAT GOOD NUTRITION CAN ALWAYS RESTORE HEALTH?

Not always. The late Dr. Max Warmbrand explained: "We are mistaken when we think of wrong diet as the *sole* cause of deficiencies. Any influence that undermines health contributes to their development: poor circulation, digestive disturbance, chronic fatigue, nervous tension and glandular disorders are all contributory factors. Deficiencies help create some of these disturbances, but in turn, these disturbances increase the deficiencies."

A change of diet alone may, and often has, restored health. If it doesn't, other adverse conditions must be corrected.

WHICH ARE BETTER: NATURAL OR SYNTHETIC VITAMINS?

Natural vitamins, if you can find them; they are rare.

WHAT IS THE DIFFERENCE BETWEEN NATURAL AND SYNTHETIC SUPPLEMENTS?

In terms of ability to correct or prevent vitamin deficiency, most chemists feel there is no structural difference between natural and synthetic vitamins. But there are actually two differences: One is that nutrients in nature do not occur alone. They are accompanied by other vitamins and minerals, which help their assimilation for body health. Synthetic vitamins are one factor standing alone (unless they are combined, in which case, they are done so by man, not by nature, and the combination is no doubt incomplete). Dr. Benjamin H. Ershoff has stated: "For all we know as our research skill and knowledge increases, we may never come to the end of the secret nutrient resources in a natural food substance."

The other little known difference between natural and synthetic substances is *proved* by chromatography, a special photographic process that pictures the difference between the substances in many foods and supplements.[9]

It is true that synthetic vitamins have been helpful during great deficiency conditions, but many therapists feel that when the deficiency begins to be corrected, synthetic vitamins continuously used in large amounts *can* be similar to drug therapy and thus likened to whipping a tired horse. Natural vitamins (condensed from natural, whole foods), which contain many interrelated nutrients, are considered safer in the long run by these therapists, for maintaining health.

HOW CAN I BE SURE THAT VITAMINS ARE NATURAL?

There are a very few manufacturers who specialize in natural vitamins. Labels do not always tell the full story. They may say that a vitamin is taken *from* a natural source, whereas it should say that the nutrient is a *whole food product* (nothing removed). Hopefully, your health food store will know which manufacturers are reliable in making available the more natural whole food vitamins.

The late Dr. Max Warmbrand said: "Vitamins and minerals are often recommended in an attempt to overcome deficiencies, but few realize that they must be derived from natural sources, otherwise the results will not be long-lasting. Many fail to realize that where the body is deficient in one element, other elements are usually lacking, too. Deficiencies occur in manifold form." Natural vitamins and minerals are a safer bet in getting *all* of them, known and unknown, into the diet.

IF YOU TAKE SUPPLEMENTS, IS IT NECESSARY TO EAT SO CAREFULLY?

Both supplements and a good diet are necessary. They work together. Food provides energy and repair materials. Supplements provide repair materials. Supplements should always be taken with meals. Since, if natural, they are food substances, they should be eaten with food. Because they are concentrated, they should usually not be taken on an empty stomach.

HOW DOES NUTRITION WORK?

Scientists have analyzed the human body and found that it is composed of sixty or more elements (some say forty, some say up to 103). Whatever the number, these elements are apparently necessary to maintain the health of the cells, glands and organs. If any of these elements are missing from your body, trouble develops. The trouble may not show up next week or next month, but sooner or later the deficiency is bound to take its toll. H. W. Holderby, M.D., has stated that at least sixty of these elements are needed; fifteen to thirty will not do the job. *All are necessary.*

If you do supply the missing or depleted nutrients, will you reverse poor health? If your problem is due to a nutritional deficiency (as is common), health can be improved. This is the whole concept of nutrition: by giving the body the necessary repair materials, it can begin to repair itself. If provided with the necessary substances before illness, it has often prevented it; if given after illness, health is usually improved. But remember that we do not claim that nutrition cures anything; it merely corrects a deficiency so that the body can help itself.

Dr. Williams summarizes: "Because every cell and tissue of our bodies needs adequate nutrition—even minute by minute—and because the different cells and tissues do not have the same needs, the problem becomes exceedingly complex. . . . If all the cells of the body receive everything they need and escape damage from poisons or infective agents, complete bodily health results. The cells do not need aspirin or other foreign chemicals. . . .

"Perhaps in the not too far distant future, many human ills will be conquered by nutritional therapy. [Meanwhile] . . . individuals need nutritional help not only to overcome illnesses that have already overtaken them, but, what is even more important, to help prevent illnesses from ever developing."

In other words, individual illnesses can be actually small signs of one major illness: malnutrition.

HOW DO YOU BEGIN YOUR IMPROVEMENT?

Since doctors are not taught nutrition in depth in medical school, you begin the improvement of your nutrition by studying yourself. No one has lived with you longer than yourself; no one knows your idiosyncrasies better. Your fingerprints are different from those of anyone else in the world. Your ailments, even though with the same names, also vary from those of others. Members of the same family, with the same parents and the same diet, can be as different from each other as night and day.

Next, you study what vitamins and minerals can accomplish—described in the remainder of this book.

Obviously, the best way to learn what vitamins and minerals you need, and how much of each is best for you, is to seek the help of a doctor who is an expert on nutrition. If you need other types of help, by all means go to the physician you need for your specific problems.

Nutritionally oriented doctors, usually self-trained, are extremely rare, but as a result of their experience gained from working with many patients they may be able to spot your deficiency quickly.

If you cannot find a nutritionally enlightened doctor the next best thing, and the thing many are forced to do, is to try to learn everything you can about nutrition yourself, and use the trial and error method in line with the scientific guidelines presented in this book. Nutrition, including natural vitamins, minerals and protein, is derived from *food,* as I have said before. If you were experimenting with drugs, which often produce dangerous side effects, it would be a different matter. Self-exploration with nutrition is admittedly slower than supervision by a nutritional physician, but if you cannot find such help, it is better than nothing. Nutritional information is given in this book to help you learn what vitamins and minerals can do and to help you cooperate with your doctor, if possible, in a mutual problem of building health.

In the event that you use this information without a doctor's approval, you are prescribing for yourself, which is your constitutional right, and I, as a reporter, do not assume responsibility. You are a law unto yourself.

In addition, hopefully, you still retain the freedom of choice to put what you wish into your own body. If your freedom of choice is, or has been, threatened, then demand the right from your congressmen. You have helped elect them and your taxes pay their salaries. They should be your spokesmen and represent your wishes.

Health is one of the greatest of all gifts. It should be cherished and protected.

Now, let us see, according to scientific research, which vitamins and minerals and foods do what.

REFERENCES

1. Beatrice Trum Hunter. *Consumer Beware!* Paperback edition. New York: Touchstone Books (Simon & Schuster), 1972.

2. Omar Garrison. *The Dictocrats' Attack on Health Foods and Vitamins.* Paperback edition. New York: Arco Publishing, 1970.

3. *Today's Health.* October, 1972.

4. Alan H. Nittler. *A New Breed of Doctor.* New York: Pyramid Communications, 1972.

5. Roger J. Williams. *You Are Extraordinary*. New York: Random House, 1967.

6. Roger J. Williams. *Biochemical Individuality*. Paperback edition. Austin, Texas: U. of Texas Press, 1969.

7. Roger J. Williams. *Nutrition Against Disease*. New York: Bantam, 1973.

8. Linda Clark. *Stay Young Longer*. Paperback edition. New York: Pyramid Communications, 1968.

9. *Let's Live*, August, 1969.

See also:

Beatrice Trum Hunter, ed. *Food and Your Health*. New Canaan, Conn.: Keats Publishing, 1974.

Charles T. McGee. *How to Survive Modern Technology*. New Canaan, Conn.: Keats Publishing, 1980.

Nutrition Research, Inc. *Nutrition Almanac*. New York: McGraw-Hill, 1979.

Jonathan V. Wright. *Dr. Wright's Book of Nutritional Therapy*. Emmaus, Pa: Rodale Press, 1979.

2
Vitamin A

There are two kinds of vitamins, fat-soluble and water-soluble. The fat-solubles are vitamins A, D, E and K; the water-solubles, the B vitamins and vitamin C. The major difference between the two types is that the fat-solubles tend to be stored in the body, whereas the water-solubles are excreted daily with liquids and therefore need to be replaced oftener. Because the fat-solubles *may* accumulate in the body, critics are quick to point out that the fat-soluble vitamins, particularly A and D, are dangerous in overdosage. But how much is too much?

In 1932, Mead, Johnson offered $15,000 as an award to anyone who could find out how much vitamin A a person needs. There were no takers, and, after thirteen years, the offer was withdrawn. Dr. Roger J. Williams states that the situation has not improved since that time. He says: "The Food and Nutrition Board, which sets up the Recommended Dietary Allowances, has thought it desirable to set down some sort of figure, and they do, but this educated guess has no foundation."

One problem is that some animals and many people

do not assimilate the vitamin A they do take. For example, vitamin A, in the form of carotene (explained later), was given to rats. Tests revealed that they absorbed only 51.5 percent of the dose, and the height of absorption was not reached until seven hours after ingestion.[1]

Another problem is that vitamin A, being a fat-soluble vitamin, *needs dietary fat to be dissolved.* A fat-free diet for reducers can be downright dangerous. A lack of fat has been found to interfere with the proper flow of bile in the gallbladder, leading to gallstones, according to a study at Bucknell University.[2] Also there are numerous books written by physicians who state that weight loss did not take place in their patients until fat in the form of vegetable oil was added to the diet.[3]

Poor liver function, alcohol, the use of mineral oil, ferrous sulfate (a form of iron), X rays, any kind of infection and even cold weather can prevent your absorbing vitamin A properly. Since there is no way of knowing how much reserve of vitamin A you have in your body, you could suddenly run out of it (if you have not been taking it regularly) without knowing it unless you recognize the symptoms of vitamin A deficiency. According to T. Keith Murphy, Ph.D., who conducted a study on the effect of a lack of vitamin A, about one out of every three people who have died of disease were deficient in vitamin A.[4]

Vitamin A is absolutely necessary for health. Be on the lookout for the following signs of a deficiency of this important vitamin:

Mucous membrane disturbances, tonsilitis, consistent cough, bronchitis (chronic), lung disorders, sinusitis, susceptibility to colds, tuberculosis, asthma, allergies and respiratory infections.

Bacterial growths

Dry skin, blackheads, whiteheads and excess wrinkles

Deep, indented ridges in fingernails

Sleeplessness

Mental confusion

Loss of balance

Peeling nails

Poor vision (particularly at dusk or at night), strong reaction to glare of any kind (such as sun or car headlights)

Soft teeth and bones (*see also* vitamin D and calcium in the next chapter)

Some types of bladder and kidney conditions, including stones, cystitis and nephritis

Disturbance of reproductive glands

Thyroid disorders, with goiter relationship

Gastritis and digestive disorders, poor appetite and diarrhea

Some types of hearing loss; loss of sense of smell

Convulsions, in some cases

Frequent fatigue and loss of pep

Vitamin A helps to protect your eyes, skin, mucous membranes, soft tissue and all linings of the digestive tract, kidneys, bladder, eyes, lungs and skin. It helps build strong bones, strong teeth and rich blood. It seems to delay senility and prolong longevity. Dr. Henry C. Sherman of Columbia University found that vitamin A added considerably to the life-span of animals and extended their youthfulness. It also helps the body to defend itself against infections.

Vitamin A contributes to good health and good teeth

in growing children. It has been found to lower cholesterol. Studies show that sufficient vitamin A is a factor needed by diabetics.[5]

Vitamin A is needed today more than ever before in history because, among other benefits it provides, it is *crucial* for protection against air pollution. Cases of emphysema and chronic bronchitis are becoming epidemic the world over, resulting in many deaths. Lung tissues are being attacked by various pollutants, including ozone, nitrogen dioxide, sulfur oxide, and all air pollutants from industrial pollution or car exhausts or radioactive fallout, as pinpointed by Dr. Ernest J. Sternglass, professor of Radiation Physics at the University of Pittsburgh, who found a direct correlation between the rise of cases of emphysema and fallout.[6] Smoking, of course, compounds the problem. But vitamin A can help.

Scientists at the Massachusetts Institute of Technology found that vitamins A and E protect lungs against air pollution. In tests at M.I.T., animals that had been deficient in vitamin A for a long time, and exhibited hard, scaly, thick lung cells, showed lung improvement within eighteen hours after the administration of vitamin A.[7]

Carl J. Reich, M.D., of Canada has had success in treating thousands cases of allergy—including bronchial asthma, chronic rhinitis and dermatitis—with vitamins A and D and bone meal. He was successful in relieving symptoms of 75 percent of 1,000 patients suffering from bronchial asthma with vitamins A and D.[8]

Dr. Eli Seifert (Albert Einstein College of Medicine) believes vitamin A activates the thymus gland which, in turn, stimulates body immunity to disease.

WHAT OTHER USES FOR VITAMIN A ARE IMPORTANT?

There are many other benefits from vitamin A. People who work in bright light and face glare (secretaries please note), watch TV a great deal, work in dim light, are exposed to the glare of sunlight, snow or many car headlights during night driving—all use up a great deal of vitamin A. Barbara Cartland, a nutrition reporter in England, believes from her experiences that fluorescent light creates a deficiency of vitamin A in the body, causing vision problems and skin blemishes. Adelle Davis agreed.

Night blindness is another common symptom of vitamin A deficiency. Pilots, both commercial and military, who do night flying are requested to take vitamin A supplements regularly.

For those who are forced to work in offices equipped with fluorescent lighting, there are two solutions. One is to take more vitamin A to compensate for the vitamin A deficiency apparently caused by fluorescents. The other is to persuade your employer to replace the fluorescent lighting with similar but *safe,* natural-type lighting tubes that fit into the same fixtures and are not too expensive. These lighting tubes have been developed as a result of the research on light by Dr. John Ott, well-known for his time-lapse photography for Walt Disney films. These tubes are called *Vita-Lite.* I feel this lighting, though hard to find, is very restful to the eyes, and it does not rob one of vitamin A. Incidentally Dr. Ott frowns on the continuous use of dark glasses. Instead, chronic glare reaction should be a warning to step up vitamin A, he believes.

Dr. Umberto Saffioti of the National Cancer Institute found that vitamin A given by mouth to hamsters exposed to cancer-causing substances prevented cancer. He also found that vitamin A in quite large amounts protected animals from cancer of the stomach, lungs and reproductive tract. These studies were confirmed by Ronald E. Davies, of the Skin and Cancer Hospital of Temple University, Philadelphia.[9] He found that animals were protected by vitamin A from skin cancer and tumors caused by a cancer-causing chemical. Those animals given vitamin A also had pinker skins and fewer wrinkles than those animals deficient in vitamin A.

Adelle Davis reported that large amounts of vitamin A taken daily cleared hundreds of large warts in one woman within four months.[10] Plantar warts have also responded to temporary massive doses of vitamin A.

Dr. Sherman found that vitamin A improved general health, resistance and vigor. A Cleveland clinic learned that a deficiency of vitamin A caused kidney stones and gallstones, while vitamin A (in cod-liver oil) dissolved many stones.

WHAT FOODS CONTAIN VITAMIN A?

Vitamin A is found in fatty fish, and fish liver oils or capsules from cod or halibut, butter fat, egg yolk, whole milk as well as in carrots, apricots, peaches, yams, yellow or orange squash, tomatoes, green peas and such green leafy vegetables as lettuce, Swiss chard, spinach and cabbage; in fact all deep green or yellow fruits and vegetables. Dairy products are another source.

WHAT IS CAROTENE?

Carotenė, sometimes called pro-vitamin A and found in foods, is a source of vitamin A. Carotene is a yellow pigment or coloring, often used for coloring cheese, margarine and other foods. Carotene is not the same as vitamin A, but once it is taken into the body it may be converted into vitamin A. For those who say we can get everything we need from our diet, carotene is one proof that this may not always be true. Carotene is very difficult for the body to utilize. Children and many adults absorb it with difficulty.[11] In fact, most healthy people have difficulty in absorbing it.

Like vitamin A, carotene needs dietary fat for absorption; it cannot dissolve in water. In addition, the cellulose in the vegetables must be broken down by cooking, chopping, chewing or juicing before carotene can be released to the body. For this reason, a cooked carrot releases more carotene than a raw carrot. Even if raw carrots are juiced, another hazard arises: much of the carotene is destroyed by oxygen when exposed to air unless the juice is drunk immediately. Therefore, it is not wise to depend upon foods for a full supply of vitamin A. Actually, carotene and vitamin A are not the same at all: vitamin A is three times more effective than the same amount of carotene.[12]

Eggs, butter and milk contain both vitamin A and carotene; the brighter the color, the greater the vitamin A content. That deep rich yellow egg yolk has more vitamin A than a pale one. Natural summer butter contains more color and thus more vitamin A than winter butter does, due to longer hours of sunlight and fresh green fodder for the cows, who convert carotene into vitamin A-rich milk and butter.

HOW ARE THE FAT-SOLUBLE VITAMINS MEASURED?

Vitamins A, D, E and K are expressed in units, known as international units, or abbreviated as "I.U."

HOW MUCH VITAMIN A SHOULD YOU USE?

This is the big question: How much vitamin A should you take daily? The amount varies with the individual, and vitamin E doubles the curative effect of A. Dr. Williams says there is no way of knowing what your own vitamin A needs are except by experimentation and observation.

Dr. Sherman recommended 20,000 I.U. daily, and Adelle Davis suggested a daily fish-liver oil capsule containing 25,000 I.U. The United States Department of Agriculture states that one cup of spinach provides 21,200 I.U. of vitamin A while only two ounces of liver furnishes 30,330 I.U. of vitamin A, so the above vitamin A recommendations do not seem too high.[13] Some people I have met can take no supplemental vitamin A at all.

Remember, vitamins A, D, E and K, all fat-soluble vitamins, cannot be absorbed without fat and bile, so those with inability to digest fat may require more vitamin A than others. There is a type of vitamin A for those who cannot tolerate fat. This type, water-dispersible A, is helpful for people who have pancreatic (fat syndrome type E) as well as gallbladder problems.

IS IT TRUE THAT VITAMIN A IN LARGE DOSES IS DANGEROUS?

There is evidence of both vitamin A and vitamin D poisoning in too large doses for some individuals, usually from prolonged use of massive doses. But Dr. Williams tells us that the variations are so great that no conclusive result has appeared. You will recall that I mentioned earlier that Dr. Williams reported the case of a man in England who took no vitamin A for twenty-two months and showed no disturbance. In another case, the woman in Pittsburgh, who took 50,000 I.U. daily, as prescribed by her doctor, also showed no disturbance. Many reported cases of vitamin A poisoning are those in which a person takes 100,000 I.U. of straight A over many months. But when the vitamin is withdrawn, the symptoms disappear within a few days to a few weeks. Each person has to experiment to find the right dosage of vitamin A for him.

WHAT ARE THE SYMPTOMS OF TOO MUCH VITAMIN A?

The symptoms include drowsiness, muscular weakness, nosebleed, headaches, blurred vision, loss of appetite, dry, scaly lips, skin rash, fretfulness, loss of energy, great desire to sleep, flamelike flashes before the eyes, dizziness, heart weakness, cramps, painful joints, tenderness over the long bones (one does not want to stand or walk) and, in a few cases, *sudden* falling out of hair. Again, let me assure you that these symptoms of *prolonged* high doses of vitamin A cease promptly within a few days or weeks, depending on how long the high dosage has been continued. A more rational dose does not produce the same symptoms described above for those people who had taken the high doses. But no one but the individual can determine the correct dosage for himself by trial and error.

Nutritional physicians say that vitamin A poisoning is both rare and curable. If you experience any of the symptoms of too much vitamin A, merely decrease the dosage until the symptoms disappear. *The Journal of the American Medical Association* states: "Withdrawal of vitamin A results in complete recovery."[14]

On the other hand, the benefits of vitamin A can range from more vigor to better vision, clearer skin, healthier hair, a relief from the deficiency symptoms listed early in this chapter, protection against and faster relief from infections and colds, and a good-to-be-alive feeling. Since vitamin A is a stimulating vitamin for some people, it should not be taken at night, for it may keep one awake. Morning is the best time to take it, preferably *after* a meal that includes some fat.

REFERENCES

1. Linda Clark. *Stay Young Longer*. Paperback edition. New York: Pyramid Communications, 1968.

2. *Ibid.*

3. Linda Clark. *Be Slim and Healthy*. Paperback edition. New Canaan, Conn.: Keats Publishing, 1972.

4. Editors of *Prevention*. "Vitamin A, Everyone's Basic Bodyguard." Emmaus, Pa.: Rodale Press, 1972.

5. *Ibid.*

6. Ernest J. Sternglass. *Low-Level Radiation*. New York: Ballantine Books, 1972.

7. *Chemical and Engineering News*. June 29, 1970.

8. *Prevention*. September, 1970, and personal communication.

9. *Cancer Research*. February, 1967.

10. Adelle Davis. *Let's Eat Right to Keep Fit*. Paperback edition. New York: New American Library, 1970.

11. *Journal of Nutrition*. October, 1967.

12. Bicknell and Prescott. *The Vitamins in Medicine*. Third edition. Milwaukee, Wis. 53201: Lee Foundation for Nutritional Research, 1962.

13. United States Department of Agriculture. *Food*

Values in Common Portions. Document No. A1B-36. Washington, D.C.: Superintendent of Documents.

14. *The Journal of the American Medical Association.* August 28, 1967.

See also:

Earl Mindell. *Earl Mindell's Vitamin Bible.* New York: Rawson Wade, 1979.

Richard A. Passwater. *Cancer and Its Nutritional Therapies.* New Canaan, Conn.: Keats Publishing, 1978.

Clifford Quick. *Sinusitis, Bronchitis and Emphysema and Their Natural Treatment.* New Canaan, Conn.: Keats Publishing, 1975.

3
Vitamin D

Vitamin D is known as the sunshine vitamin because its main source is the sun. Ultraviolet light from the sun transforms the ergosterol (an oily substance) on the skin into vitamin D, which is, in turn, transferred through the skin into the blood stream.

Vitamin D in the blood increases the absorption of calcium and phosphorus in the intestines, which promotes the normal growth of bones, prevents rickets and maintains a normal calcium-phosphorus balance, vitality and good health. It is obvious that people who spend more time outdoors look better and feel healthier than those who spend too much time indoors. The main reason for the difference is vitamin D.

Vitamin D can do some surprising things for you. It can protect you against muscular weakness and be the guardian for your bones. It can help you to assimilate the calcium you take into your body, and thus help regulate your heart. If you do not have enough calcium in your body, the parts that need it most (such as teeth and bones) will rob Peter to pay Paul by withdrawing it from other areas where it is also needed. Or it may be taken from the bones of another area. For example, if your heart begins to flutter (a process called fibrillation) because your calcium level has become too low, calcium can be borrowed from your bones to answer the distress signal from your heart.

Vitamin D must be on hand to help this emergency borrowing process. If vitamin D is lacking, the heart's SOS may not be answered.

Two hundred and forty-eight executives, averaging forty years of age, were regular participants of a physical conditioning program at NASA's Manned Spacecraft Center, Houston, Texas. During their exercises, eighty-four of these men developed heart irregularities, but none of them were found to have detectable heart disease. Although no conclusive results were announced, there was conjecture that the men may have had too little vitamin D, or calcium, or both.[1]

Another surprising use of vitamin D is that of relieving nearsightedness. Arthur A. Knapp, M.D., a New York ophthalmologist, believes that nearsightedness is a manifestation of vitamin D deficiency. He gave a group of patients large doses of vitamin D with calcium, for a period of five to twenty-eight months. Nearsightedness was decreased in more than 33 percent and halted in 17 percent. Dr. Knapp, although he has not concluded sufficient research on cataracts, believes that they, too, may result from vitamin D and calcium deficiencies. At least animals kept on diets deficient in vitamin D and calcium invariably develop cataracts, he states.[2] (For other causes of cataracts see *Handbook of Natural Remedies for Common Ailments* by Linda Clark.)

People who are cooped up indoors in colder climates become paler as winter continues. Even office workers in warm climates are sun-starved. Since vitamin D occurs in so few foods, and most people do not take vitamin D supplements, indoor workers may not get any at all. Student nurses, for example, working inside during the sun-lit hours in Michigan, were found to have no vitamin D in their bloodstreams. Yet factory workers who ate their lunches outdoors acquired sufficient sun on the skin of the face, neck and arms, to provide a useful amount of vitamin D for better health.

Sunshine has been found to help the skin synthesize vitamin D at the rate of 18 I.U. per square centimeter of skin in three hours.[3]

Animals bask in the sun for a limited amount of time to collect vitamin D on their coats. People who are sun-starved are not so wise. During their vacation, they go to the opposite extreme and bake themselves to a crisp, which does more harm than good. And even if they anoint themselves with oil because their skins have dried out, after sun tanning they take a shower and wash off all the vitamin D they have accumulated. Too much sun is now acknowledged as a major cause of skin cancer, so moderation is necessary.

But there are other reasons for a lack of vitamin D. Even if people spend time outdoors in warmer climates, the sun cannot penetrate clothes, fog or smog to reach the skin and manufacture enough vitamin D. It was formerly thought that only children needed vitamin D. Doctors advised mothers to get their children out in the sunshine during the summer and to give them cod liver oil in the winter to prevent or cure rickets. This therapy is as old as the hills. Now we know that everybody needs vitamin D the year round. And, the need increases with age. Since this vitamin helps to make strong bones, the fragile, brittle bones of the elderly may be due as much to a lack of vitamin D as to a lack of calcium, with which vitamin D cooperates. The solution to the problem of vitamin D deficiency is to take it in supplement form. Many experts advise no more than 400 I.U. vitamin D daily.

WHAT ARE THE SYMPTOMS OF VITAMIN D DEFICIENCY?

Paleness due to lack of exposure to sun
Fragile bones in adults, rickets in children (causes bowed legs, knock-knees, sway back, protruding abdomen), and osteoporosis
Arthritis (in some cases)
Soft teeth, cavities and pyorrhea (gum disturbance)
Nervousness, irritability and tension
Sensitivity to pain
Insomnia
Tuberculosis type of infection of skin and psoriasis (in some cases)
Nearsightedness (in some cases) and conjunctivitis
Muscle spasms or cramps
Bronchitis
Nosebleed and some other types of hemorrhage
Restlessness and fast heart beat
Delayed healing

You will recognize many of these symptoms as the same as those of calcium and vitamin A deficiency. Vitamin D is a partner of calcium, as well as of vitamin A. Vitamin D, like A, is found in fish-liver oils, needs fat and bile for absorption when taken by mouth, and is measured in supplements in international units.

CAN VITAMIN D BE TOXIC?

Vitamin D is the only other vitamin, beside vitamin A, that can be toxic when taken in too large doses. Excessive doses of vitamin D overmobilize the calcium (and phosphorus) out of the tissues, producing the opposite effects of a normal dose. When vitamin D is taken in too large doses, it is stored in the liver, and keeps accumulating. It is not eliminated like the B or other water-soluble vitamins.

WHAT ARE THE SYMPTOMS OF VITAMIN D POISONING?

Nausea
Loss of appetite
Vomiting
Cramps
Diarrhea or constipation
Tingling in fingers and toes
Dizziness
Excess calcification of bones
Hardening of the arteries (a type of calcification)
Abdominal pain
Fatigue or weakness
Intense thirst
Confused memory
Headaches or tenderness to pressure on head
Dislike of noise
Pain in jaws
Tender teeth, joints and muscles

Now, please note that these same symptoms can also be caused by *other factors*. But read the labels of your other supplements and beware of getting too much. The question is: How much is too much? Again, as in the case of vitamin A, nobody knows. Even the Food and Nutrition Board gives a realistic answer to this one. They say: "There is no recommendation for vitamin D for adults over twenty-two years of age since there is no data available upon which to base such a recommendation."

Doses ranging from 400 I.U. daily upward have been safety-tested. But again, there is such a wide margin of individual difference that 400 I.U. may not be enough for some people..

Dr. Roger J. Williams says:

"There is no vitamin that cannot be administered safely at a level ten times that of the supposed need."[4]

R. W. Smith, Ph.D., and associates have reported in the *American Journal of Clinical Nutrition* that adults can benefit from 2,500 to 5,000 I.U. vitamin D daily. In older people, stress, illness and aging may use up even more vitamin D.

However, when vitamin D has been increased to 3,900 I.U. daily, ten times more calcium was assimilated by the body.[5]

It is possible that 50,000 I.U. might bring on severe vitamin D poisoning. One study made by the National Institutes of Health on people who were extremely sensitive to vitamin D found that it took only 10,000 I.U. per day to produce toxicity.

Toxicity of vitamin D has been found preventable by generous amounts of vitamin A, choline (a B vitamin) and vitamin C.[6]

Meanwhile, a moderate exposure to sunshine is always a good idea for everyone. Don't overdo it.

There are few foods containing vitamin D: egg yolk, fish, fish-liver oil (halibut-liver oil is the richest in this vitamin), and milk. Thus one usually needs to fall back upon a supplement to supply it. And here lies a hazard. A probable rational daily dose may be 1,500 I.U., with 2,000 I.U. per day for greater needs. But if you should be taking a multiple vitamin capsule that contains this amount, and should decide you want to double the dosage, you are doubling the amount of vitamin D, which may not be safe. *So read your labels.*

WHAT TYPES OF VITAMIN D ARE AVAILABLE IN SUPPLEMENTS?

Vitamin D comes naturally from sunlight, but as we have seen exposure to the sun should not be overdone, nor should it be washed off immediately after sunning until it has had a chance to penetrate the body. In supplement form there is no vitamin D-1, only vitamin D-2 and D-3. Vitamin D-3 is the natural form. Vitamin D-2 is known as calciferol, made by irradiating a substance called ergosterol. It is synthetic, and was the culprit used many years ago in drop form for babies. The trouble was that the mothers, told by their doctors to give a specific number of drops of this substance, decided if some is good, more is better, and gave babies this synthetic vitamin D by the teaspoonful instead of the prescribed drops, resulting in serious trouble for the children.

I use vitamin D-3 (the natural form) only.

There is much controversy about how much vitamin D is safe as well as effective. Some investigators and even doctors recommend huge amounts but only once a week. (This is because vitamin D and other fat-soluble vitamins are stored in the body and too much may eventually become toxic.)

Years ago Dr. Agnes Fay Morgan, the ex-Dean Emeritus of the Nutrition Department of the University of California, Berkeley, conducted in-depth studies on dogs and found that no more than 400 units of vitamin D on a daily basis were safe. (This amount is also accepted by the present RDAs.)

I have vast respect for Dr. Morgan and her work and as a result, I, personally, take only 400 I.U. of vitamin D-3 daily. Although other nutritionists claim that if you take certain other vitamins at the same time as the larger doses of vitamin D, the toxicity risk is lowered, I am afraid to take the chance. Also the computation becomes too complicated for me in these already over-complex times.

Vitamin D is extremely important because it activates the two small parathyroid glands (located close to the thyroid). These little glands help the body to assimilate calcium.

One of the recent rediscovered findings is that when the parathyroids have been removed from dogs, their calcium assimilation ceases abruptly. But the research of Dr. Charles Bayle, of Paris, France, showed that if spleen tissue were given to the dogs, as a substitute for the missing parathyroids, calcium manufacture was resumed instantly.[7] Spleen tissue is available from health stores if you feel your parathyroid function is inadequate. Meanwhile, to keep your parathyroids working, look to vitamin D!

Vitamin D poisoning is something to watch for, not fear. The results after withdrawing vitamin D are fast; symptoms may disappear within a few days. It, like vitamin A, can be controlled, particularly if it is taken separately (as in a vitamin A/D combination) rather than in a multiple vitamin preparation.

The best and safest way I know to get both vitamin A

and vitamin D is by taking cod-liver oil. This has been taken for years without adverse effects. Some of you may shudder and insist that you can't "stomach" it. I sympathize. I have given it to my children from babyhood without batting an eye, as my pediatrician told me to, and the children took it happily without flinching. They, in turn, have given it to their children, also with no fuss. But not I; I can't bear the odor or the taste of cod-liver oil. Yet I have learned a method of taking it so that I actually relish it.

I use the mint-flavored cod-liver oil and this is how I take it: I keep the bottle refrigerated, together with a special empty container, such as a small jar or wide-mouthed bottle reserved for this purpose. On an empty stomach, first thing in the morning or last thing before bedtime, I put two tablespoons of cold fruit juice of some kind in the empty container, add one tablespoon of the cold mint-flavored cod-liver oil, and shake the two together—as in a cocktail shaker—and drink the mix directly from the container, which I return, unwashed, to the refrigerator. The mixture is delightful.

I do not wash the container because once a spoon or container is coated with the oil and is washed with dishes, it smells up everything with which it comes in contact. It is easier to use the same container again and again. If it gets too strong, throw it away and replace it with a fresh one. The reason I take it on an empty stomach is that one investigator insists it doesn't put on weight when taken this way. This may be right or wrong, but I do it. I do know that I have seen dry skin and hair take on a new sheen within two weeks after beginning the cod-liver oil routine.

There are a few people who complain that cod-liver oil repeats on them and they burp it at intervals. In this case, one doctor has suggested that one may use the cod-liver oil in capsules, beginning with one per day and working up to eight daily. He feels that this conditions the individual to it and prevents the repeating or burping. And if one does not get much sun in summer, it is wise to continue this cod-liver oil procedure the year round. It is a happy medium route; one doesn't develop a deficiency of vitamin D, nor run the risk of getting too much.

REFERENCES

1. Jane Kinderlehrer. "Heart and Nerves Need Vitamin D." *Prevention.* September, 1972.

2. Ruth Adams. *The Complete Home Guide to All the Vitamins.* New York: Larchmont Books, 1972.

3. *The Medical Journal of Australia.* August 24, 1968.

4. Roger J. Williams. *Nutrition Against Disease.* Paperback edition. New York: Bantam, 1973.

5. *American Journal of Diseases of Children.* Vol. 67, p. 265, 1944.

6. *Archives of Diseases of Childhood.* Vol. 35, p. 385, 1960.

7. Linda Clark. "The Spleen." *Let's Live* Magazine. February, 1980, p. 121.

See also: The Complete Book of Vitamins. Emmaus, Pa.: Rodale Press, 1966.

Bicknell and Prescott. *The Vitamins in Medicine.* Third Edition. Milwaukee, Wis. 53201: Lee Foundation for Nutritional Research, 1962.

Arthur Alexander Knapp. "Prevention of Blindness." *New Dynamics of Preventive Medicine,* vol. 2. Leon Pomeroy, ed. Miami, Fla. Symposia Specialists, 1974.

4
The Vitamin E Story

Vitamin E, originally isolated from wheat germ oil, is perhaps our most important vitamin because, among other things, it helps to keep our hearts in good working order, a function essential to life itself.

There is proof of this good effect of vitamin E on hearts. When the Minnesota Agricultural Experiment Station found cattle suddenly dropping dead from no apparent cause, extensive tests finally pinpointed the reason: they had been deprived of the vitamin E rations in their feed and had died of heart disease. When vitamin E was restored to their feed, the deaths from heart disease stopped.[1]

Most people are deprived of vitamin E in their food today, just as those cattle were, and this is no doubt a major cause of the nation's alarming increase of heart disease. Vitamin E, which was formerly available in wholegrain flour, breads and cereals as well as in natural oils, is now lost in refining. Wheat germ, the richest source known of vitamin E, has been removed from the bread and cereal because of its fragility; it will not keep long on the grocer's shelf. So the nation, if not the world, is being subjected to the dietary loss of this vitamin so necessary in their diet.

For those who point an accusing finger toward saturated fats and even sugar, both of which no doubt do play a role in undermining the heart, Wilfrid E. Shute, M.D., one of the two outstanding physicians in the world who has treated heart disease successfully with vitamin E, makes an impressive statement: "Prior to the removal of wheat germ with its vitamin E, there were no cases of coronary thrombosis. Now it is one of the nation's major killers."

Dr. Shute continues: "Heart attacks have been blamed on stress and strain, on overexertion, on the fast pace of modern living, on soft drinking water, on hard drinking water and, of course, on diets rich in animal fats. Yet, with each and every one, it can be shown that the same condition was present in the lives of all or many people prior to 1900, but did not cause coronary thrombosis. There is an explanation so simple that it would be automatically suspect had its truth not already been demonstrated in clinical practice of more than twenty years involving many thousands of patients. I have found vitamin E a superb anti-thrombin (clot dissolver) in the bloodstream. Flour milling underwent a great change around the turn of the century. The vitamin E in the diet was greatly reduced and with the loss of this natural anti-thrombin, coronary thrombosis appeared on the scene."[2]

Dr. Shute is quick to admit that coronary thrombosis is not the only form of heart disease, but it is by far the major cause of more than one million deaths a year in the United States alone. And even in other forms of heart disease, vitamin E has proved useful, both for prevention and treatment.

Before we learn how vitamin E works, not only to protect hearts, but for treating many other conditions as well, you should know that the path of vitamin E in the national dietary has not been smooth. Controversy over vitamin E began to rage in this country soon after it was discovered in 1922.[3] Even twenty years later, the FDA and the AMA refused to acknowledge that it was useful at all and ignored abundant evidence of its success with both animals and people in nearly every other country in the world. Not only was the evidence for this wonderful vitamin ignored, it was belittled, called absolutely worthless, and the FDA refused to list it as essential to human health. The reason was that some doctors who had tried it with their patients used too small a dose either for the individual or for the type of disease, for which vitamin E has been so successful when used properly.

Meanwhile, in 1945, the two Canadian brothers, Evan V. Shute, M.D., a gynecologist and obstetrician, now deceased, and Wilfrid E. Shute, M.D., a heart specialist, began to use vitamin E in heart and other disturbances with brilliant success.

Here are some examples:[4]

One man, a wheelchair angina invalid, who experienced excruciating pains just carrying on a conversation, was treated by the Shute brothers in their clinic in London, Ontario, Canada. This man was freed from his wheelchair by massive doses of vitamin E: as a result he could fish all day, play bridge until midnight and enjoy nine holes of golf.

Another angina patient, seventy-one years old, suffered from extreme pain after the slightest exertion. Vitamin E made it possible for him to do heavy work at a tannery.

A man of twenty-six, stricken with rheumatic fever

during childhood, was able, because of vitamin E, to work in a foundry.

A musician of fifty-two, with recurrent attacks of coronary thrombosis over a period of five years, did not spend another day in bed after taking vitamin E.

The Shute brothers had successfully treated more than 10,000 patients by 1955 (now more than 30,000 cases) for coronary thrombosis, angina and rheumatic heart disease. They learned that vitamin E apparently increases the oxygen supply to the heart and other muscles and it dissolves clots if they are fresh, or bypasses sites of older clots or vascular blockage, thus increasing the circulation. It was not unusual for their patients to recover from a heart attack, get out of bed and return to mowing lawns within weeks after their attack. And it is not unusual for patients on the proper dose of vitamin E to maintain their useful heart function for many years without any returning symptoms.

Finally the public and many scientists demanded that the FDA accept vitamin E as essential in the human diet, and so, reluctantly, in 1959, the FDA was forced to recognize the vitamin and give it credit. However, only the need—not the daily requirement—was acknowledged. On the list of the dietary allowances set up by the Food and Nutrition Board of the National Academy of Sciences the usual Recommended Dietary Allowance of vitamin E is shockingly low.

In fact, the Shute brothers, and others who use vitamin E successfully, believe this amount far too low to bring good results at all. But most orthodox physicians still believe the original propaganda against vitamin E and do not prescribe even the minimum. Yet, but for its use in proper amounts, many people would not be alive today.

HOW MUCH VITAMIN E SHOULD ONE TAKE?

Dr. Evan Shute said: "As our experience has increased, our doses of alpha tocopherol (the type of vitamin E used by these doctors) have risen in parallel."

If there is something like a physiological dam that prevents the vitamin E from getting to the tissues, then the idea is to raise the level of vitamin E until it runs over the dam. Dr. Shute continued: "Our success with the procedure has been marked. Notably in persistent anginas, arteriosclerotic conditions, chronic leg ulcers and chronic phlebitis.

"Half a dose of alpha tocopherol does not do half a job, as we pointed out years ago. One either uses the proper dose for that patient and his particular condition, or one is not using anything. Too small a dose is equivalent to half-treating a diabetic . . . if one is in doubt it is (with two exceptions) safer to overtreat than to undertreat. Let us emphasize this point. If you use vitamin E, use enough."[5]

The Shute Institute used, for various people and various conditions, doses usually ranging from 300 to 2,400 I.U. daily, depending on the circumstances. Without a doctor to guide you, you must feel your way and learn by trial as the Shutes have done. Starting out with 100 or 200 I.U. daily, and gradually increasing it by the week, the dose for the individual is usually established when optimum results are felt, but before any side effects are experienced. As the Shute brothers stated, this must be done for each individual. Obviously, the way to determine the correct dosage is with the help of a doctor who is conversant with vitamin E therapy. If this is impossible, read *every word* of *Vitamin E for Ailing and Healthy Hearts* by Wilfrid E. Shute and Harald J. Taub or *The*

Complete, Updated Vitamin E Book by Wilfrid E. Shute be
fore embarking on your experiment. Or take the book to
your doctor. Many doctors are reading them and their
patients are benefiting as a result.[6]

Dr. Evan V. Shute, internationally renowned for his
more than thirty years of experience with vitamin E,
believed that there is a small minority who cannot take
50 or 100 or even 300 I.U. a day. He said: "We think
that the average normal male should have about 600 a
day and the average female about 400 a day."[7]

According to Dr. Wilfrid E. Shute, if overactivity is
experienced, vitamin E should be omitted for two full
days only, before starting at a slightly lower dose, since
vitamin E leaves the blood stream entirely after three
days. There is a test for a deficiency of vitamin E. Since
anemia can be caused by a vitamin E deficiency, the
speed with which the red blood cells are destroyed in the
body is used as a test for the deficiency of the vitamin.[8]

IS THERE DANGER IN TAKING TOO MUCH VITAMIN E?

Yes, in two conditions: high blood pressure and rheumatic heart conditions. If too much vitamin E is given at
first to hypertension (high blood pressure) patients, it
sends the pressure up. In this case, Dr. Wilfrid Shute
says: "The initial dose should be no more than 90 I.U.,
perhaps less, per day for a month. For the second month,
it is increased to 120 I.U. daily and for the third month,
150 I.U."[9] For rheumatic heart patients, he recommends
an equivalent dosage, rarely going over 300 I.U. per day.
He warns: "Starting a victim of chronic rheumatic heart
disease on a high dose can lead to rapid deterioration or
death."[10]

A German physician gave vitamin E to 100 patients to reduce high blood pressure. However, he used very low dosages of the vitamin. For most patients with high blood pressure, many physicians do not advise taking more than 800 I.U. daily.[11]

VITAMIN E ANTAGONISTS

According to Dr. Wilfrid Shute there are several substances that interfere with, or even cancel out vitamin E in the body. They are *inorganic* iron, estrogen (female hormones) and chlorine.

There are easy solutions to these problems. If you are taking inorganic iron and/or female hormones, merely take vitamin E twelve hours distant from the antagonists. You could take the vitamin E in the morning, for example, and the iron and female hormones at night. As for chlorine (Dr. H. M. Sinclair of England believes its presence in water destroys vitamin E in the body), this is easily remedied, too. Either boil your water, or leave it in an open container overnight to help the chlorine evaporate. The water can then be refrigerated for drinking purposes.

Because the increase of polyunsaturated fats or oils in the diet increases the rate of oxidation of vitamin E, *the more unsaturated fats or oils added, the more vitamin E is necessary.*

Ruth Adams, researcher and author, states: "Another reason for a possible shortage of vitamin E [in our diet] is that many of the foods we eat today have been frozen."[12]

IN WHAT FOODS IS VITAMIN E FOUND?

Vitamin E is plentiful in most vegetable oils, with safflower oil and wheat germ the richest sources. It is also found in all seeds, eggs, leafy vegetables, beef liver, meat, milk, molasses, nuts (preferably raw), peanuts and legumes (soybeans, peas and beans).

The richest sources of vitamin E are the vegetable oils (unrefined) and unrefined cereal products, especially wheat germ, and eggs. Of the oils, crude wheat germ oil contains the highest amount of vitamin E; soybean oil is next. Although cottonseed oil is not particularly high in vitamin E, it is often used as a source, or combined with other oils such as soybean oil. However, some of these sources create a problem for those who take vitamin E.

IS IT TRUE THAT SOME PEOPLE ARE ALLERGIC TO SOME FORMS OF VITAMINS?

Statistics show that there are two top-ranking allergens (sources of allergies) in this country: chocolate and wheat. Those who are allergic to wheat could also be allergic to vitamin E derived from wheat germ oil. One company makes a vitamin E product from soybean and cottonseed oil, thus bypassing wheat germ, but this combination raises another serious problem. As verified by the Department of Agriculture in Los Angeles, cottonseed oil, though reasonably high in vitamin E and protein, is said to contain an allergen of its own of which many people are unaware.

Furthermore, also confirmed by the same office of the Department of Agriculture, the use of poisons and pesticides on cotton is unrestricted; thus the oil apparently usually contains the hydrocarbon pesticides. For this reason, many experts believe that vitamin E should not be combined with or derived from cottonseed oil.

What to do for a vitamin E allergy? It is hard to say. Some people who are allergic to vitamin E in oils (including wheat-germ oil) may take it in the dry form. At least one company makes it available in this form in capsules. It is also available in tablets. Dr. Wilfrid E. Shute wrote me that though they now use the natural vitamin E, their original research and success were achieved by the use of synthetic vitamin E. So, if worse comes to worst, the synthetic may be the only solution for those who suspect an allergy from other sources.

One researcher has found that older people often respond better to the succinate form of vitamin E. Dr. Shute suggests that either the succinate or the acetate can be used by those who are allergic to wheat and vitamin E derived from it.

WHAT TYPES OF VITAMIN E EXIST?

Vitamin E is named "tocopherol," a chemical name derived from the Greek. It was so named because it was originally studied in connection with fertility (and is still considered a "fertility" vitamin). The first factor discovered was alpha tocopherol. Since then, newer ones have been discovered and isolated. Each new tocopherol is given the next name in the Greek alphabet. To date, there are—in addition to alpha tocopherol—beta, gamma, delta and epsilon tocopherols. Usually a vitamin E label states that the product includes alpha tocopherol only, and the Shute brothers have always used this exclusively. But mixed tocopherols are now available, too. There is a belief in some quarters that the other tocopherols may eventually prove as important, in their own way, as alpha tocopherol.

Vitamin E, like the other oily vitamins, is labeled in international units. Even if a vitamin E product is labeled as "mixed tocopherols," the potency is based upon the amount of alpha tocopherol included, and the mixed tocopherols are extra. Vitamin E usually comes in potencies of 100, 200 or even higher I.U. Even if the product contains mixed tocopherols, the label means that there is that much alpha tocopherol in the product. One company makes it crystal clear. Its label states: "Vitamin E, contains 100 I.U. of alpha tocopherol, plus 50 mg of beta, gamma and delta tocopherols." Some people prefer these mixed tocopherols.

The advantage of mixed tocopherol products is that they have greater antioxidant activity due to the presence of the beta, delta and gamma tocopherols with the alpha tocopherol. An explanation of the word antioxidant is a substance which can prevent undesirable forms of oxygen in the body from causing damage to body cells and causing fat rancidity. Since vitamin E protects against fat rancidity in the body, we need more vitamin E when higher amounts of dietary fats and oils (even cod liver oil) are consumed.

WHAT IS THE BEST TYPE OF VITAMIN E TO TAKE?

Many people prefer not only the mixed tocopherols, which represent the whole vitamin E family, but natural vitamin E instead of synthetic. Is the natural vitamin E really better? It appears to depend upon the person taking it. For example, in early stages of whooping cough, vitamin E was found to be a help. Natural vitamin E proved to be active; synthetic E did not.[13]

HOW CAN I TELL WHICH E IS NATURAL?

According to the J. R. Carlson Laboratories, Inc., in Illinois, specialists in natural vitamin E, the letter or letters preceding the name on the vitamin E label tell the story: "d" means natural; "dl" synthetic.

NATURAL VITAMIN E PREPARATIONS MARKETED TODAY READ:	SYNTHETIC VITAMIN E PREPARATIONS MARKETED TODAY READ:
d-alpha tocopherol	dl-alpha tocopherol
d-alpha tocopheryl acetate	dl-alpha tocopheryl acetate
d-alpha tocopheryl-succinate	dl-alpha tocopheryl-succinate (from Europe)
mixed tocopherols	

WHAT IS ACETATE? WHAT IS SUCCINATE?

Acetate and succinate are organic substances naturally found in our bodies. When combined with vitamin E they provide resistance against oxidation (rancidity) and spoilage.

WHAT IS THE DIFFERENCE BETWEEN THE SPELLINGS OF TOCOPHEROL AND TOCOPHERYL?

The "y" spelling is used when the name of the ester (acetate or succinate) follows the word "alpha." Otherwise, the "o" spelling is used.

WHAT TYPE OF VITAMIN E IS BEST?

Some people have trouble digesting oils. There is a dry E in capsule or tablet form. In addition to its ability to be better digested by those who have fat-digestion problems, the dry E is often coupled with pectin, which is used as an emulsifier and speeds up the digestion of vitamin E. However, those who take the oily vitamin E are found to have more vitamin E in the bloodstream several hours later. A new vitamin E, put out by a natural vitamin company, now contains vitamin E in wheat-germ oil with lecithin as an emulsifier. There are also water-dispersible forms of vitamin E. One of these comes in capsules, another in drops, yielding 10 I.U. of vitamin E per drop. This should be a boon for babies and small children.

However, some nutritionists believe that we should not avoid oily products, even if we have an oil- or fat-digestion problem. Apparently we do not assimilate our minerals without oil and the gallbladder must have oil in order to function. One suggestion is that we are better off, nutritionally, taking the oily vitamins but also taking digestive enzymes such as hydrochloric acid, pancreatic enzymes and perhaps bile salts, to help digest the oils, than avoiding dietary fats. These are available in health stores.

It takes a tankful of oil to make one cup of natural vitamin E. The supply of natural vitamin E is limited and more expensive than many vitamins. Most multiple vitamin supplements contain very little vitamin E, therefore it generally needs to be added separately to your supplement program.

IS IT BETTER TO TAKE WHEAT-GERM OIL TO OBTAIN VITAMIN E THAN TO TAKE VITAMIN E CAPSULES OR TABLETS?

You would have to take ten teaspoons of wheat-germ oil in order to get 100 I.U. of vitamin E. Since the Shutes believed 400 to 600 I.U. the minimum dosage for the average woman and man, this would take a lot of wheat-germ oil, which is an excellent product for many, but the flavor and texture at least in large amounts turns many people off.

WHAT ARE THE BENEFITS OF TAKING VITAMIN E?

There have been at least 3,800 medical and scientific studies proving the success of vitamin E and the fact that some sixty ailments have been associated with a deficiency of vitamin E. According to these sources as well as the findings of the Doctors Shute, vitamin E:

Supplies oxygen to the muscles (the heart is a muscle) and guides oxygen to the cells.

Prevents rancidity when added to other substances. It is often added to vitamin A for this reason.

Is a natural anticoagulant. It can dissolve blood clots safely and turn itself off when the blood has reached the desired consistency, whereas anticlotting drugs (heparin and dicumarol) can become dangerous by overthinning the blood.

Can also permeate the tiny capillaries and bring nourishment to them. For the eyes, for example, this is invaluable.

Other miracles accomplished by vitamin E:

Protects lungs against air pollution, as established by Dr. E. L. Robert Stokstad, University of California, Berkeley. Also used for the same purpose together with vitamin A as tested by M.I.T. scientists (see chapter on vitamin A)

Prevents ulcers[14]

Can prevent: wasting and weakness of muscle tissue; disorders of reproductive glands; miscarriages; sterility in animals, men and women; stillbirths; spontaneous abortions; menopause symptoms, including hot flashes and sweating.[15] (A farm journal in Rumania reported a study in which vitamin E plus vitamin A were given to seventy-seven sterile cows: 70 percent of them then conceived.)[16]

Has helped (in some cases) cerebral palsy, Parkinson's disease, and muscular dystrophy, particularly when combined with other nutritional substances[17,18]

Prevents or relieves: coronary heart disease, angina pectoris, varicose veins, indolent ulcers, thrombosis, phlebitis (clots), Buerger's disease, kidney disease, and gangrene and retinal changes in diabetes mellitus[19]

Protects against flu and used topically is useful for certain skin diseases, rashes and scars.

Is an outstanding treatment for burns. Before and after pictures of a man severely burned on his face and arms in an industrial explosion show the charred flesh, and, only three weeks later, as a result of taking vitamin E internally and applying it externally in the form of an ointment, the flesh changed back to near normal. The skin eventually healed without any disfiguration. (This is one of the most spectacular evidences of vitamin E healing ever reported.)[20,21]

Is used for some eye diseases[22]

Lowers cholesterol far exceeding claims for a low cholesterol diet[23]

Improves circulation and resistance to cold, and helps cold hands and feet[24]

Aids protein assimilation[25]

Relieves leg cramps[26]

Retards aging[27]

In one case of diabetes mellitus, brought blood sugar

to normal with 200 I.U. of mixed tocopherols daily, within
three months[28]

Is used for painful legs[29]

Has prevented calcification of aorta and kidneys[30]

Has counteracted liver changes in rats intoxicated
with carbon tetrachloride[31]

Increases mobility and breathing[31]

Has eliminated loss of muscle tissue in monkeys who
could not right themselves when laid on their sides; vitamin E brought complete recovery within two to three
weeks[32]

Heals scar tissue produced by X rays[33]

Can be rubbed on stings, insect bites and burns[34]

There are more uses of vitamin E coming to our
attention. But with its unique accomplishments thus far,
who can deny its miracle ability?

CONTRA-INDICATIONS FOR VITAMIN E FOR SOME PEOPLE

As I have said before, some intolerance to vitamin
E may be due to the type of E the person is taking.
Vitamin E was originally isolated from wheat germ.
Meanwhile, wheat and wheat products have been found
to be a problem for many people the world over. One
medical clinic and several independent physicians confirm this. For those who are intolerant to wheat, symptoms can vary, differing with the individual. Fatigue,
flatulence (gas), rashes, elevated blood pressure and other
problems have been reported. Celiac disease and multiple
sclerosis seem to follow a wheat intolerance, due to gluten, a wheat ingredient.[35] Many wheat-intolerant people
realize there is something wrong with them but do not

connect the ailment with the possible cause: wheat. Wheat germ, recommended highly as an excellent food, can cause, for some, rashes and other more serious side-effects. For the same reason many people are disturbed by vitamin E *if* it is derived from wheat germ oil.

Fortunately there is a solution to this problem. Vitamin E does not have to depend upon wheat germ any longer. Higher concentrations of it are found in unrefined vegetable oils, nuts and whole raw seeds. So if you are intolerant to vitamin E, read your label. If the source is wheat germ oil, select a vitamin E from another type of oil. Natural vitamin E is also available in a number of vegetable oils. It bears repeating that *the more polyunsaturated oils are taken, the more vitamin E is needed.*[36]

REFERENCES

1. Gullickson and Calverly. "Cardiac Failure on Vitamin-Free Rations as Revealed by Electrocardiogram." *Science,* p. 312. October 3, 1946.

2. Wilfrid E. Shute with Harald J. Taub. *Vitamin E for Ailing and Healthy Hearts.* Paperback edition. New York: Jove Books (BJ Publishing Group), 1972.

3. *Annotated Bibliography of Vitamin E.* New York (150 Broadway, New York 10007): National Vitamin Foundation.

4. J. D. Ratcliffe. "For Heart Disease, Vitamin E." *Coronet,* October, 1948.

5. "Natural Food Supplements." *Prevention,* May, 1971, p. 86.

6. Wilfrid E. Shute with Harald J. Taub. *op. cit.*

7. Linda Clark, *Stay Young Longer.* Paperback edition. New York: Pyramid Communications, 1968.

8. Wilfrid E. Shute with Harald J. Taub. *op. cit.* Wilfrid E Shute. *The Complete Updated Vitamin E Book.* New Canaan, Conn.: Keats Publishing Inc., 1975.

9. *Ibid.*

10. *Ibid.*

11. Ruth Adams and Frank Murray. *Vitamin E— Wonder Worker of the 70's?* Paperback edition. New York: Manor Books, 1972.

12. Ruth Adams. *The Complete Home Guide to All the Vitamins.* New York: Larchmont Press, 1972.

13. Aillaud and Raybaud. *Marseille Medicine,* Vol. 107, No. 6, 1970.

14. *Annotated Bibliography of Vitamin E, op. cit.*

15. Wilfrid E. Shute and Harald J. Taub, *op. cit.*

16. Ruth Adams and Frank Murray, *op. cit.*

17. *Nutritional Abstracts and Reviews,* January, 1957, p. 65.

18. Ruth Adams and Frank Murray, *op. cit.*

19. Report of the Symposium on Vitamin E Conducted by the West German Federal Society of Nutrition, 1965.

20. Adelle Davis. *Let's Get Well.* Paperback edition. New York: New American Library, 1972.

21. Marvel Berst. "The Better Treatment of Burns." *Prevention.* January, 1973.

22. Adelle Davis, *op. cit.*

23. *Journal of the American Pediatrics Society.* 1971, Vol. 19, pp. 962-969.

24. Ruth Adams and Frank Murray, *op. cit.*

25. *Ibid.*

26. Ruth Adams. *op. cit.*

27. *Journal of Gerontology.* July, 1961.

28. J. I. Rodale and Staff. *The Complete Book of Vita-*

mins. Emmaus, Pa.: Rodale Books, 1966.

29. *Prevention.* November, 1970, p. 75.

30. *Nutrition Abstracts and Reviews.* July, 1964. Abstract No. 3921.

31. *Nutrition Abstracts and Reviews.* April, 1960. Abstract No. 1933.

32. *Nutrition Abstracts and Reviews.* January, 1957. p. 65.

33. *Modern Nutrition.* June, 1951.

34. *Prevention.* October, 1960, p. 38.

35. Hilda Cherry Hills. *Good Food, Gluten Free.* New Canaan, Conn.: Keats Publishing, 1976.

36. M. K. Horwitt. *Vitamins and Hormones* 201: 541-58.

See also:

Jack Joseph Challem. "Vitamin E: Better for Burns and Scars." *Health Quarterly,* vol. 6, no. 2.

Lawrence Galton. *Medical Advances.* New York: Crown Publishers, Inc., 1977.

Evan V. Shute. *The Heart and Vitamin E.* New Canaan, Conn.: Keats Publishing, 1977.

Wilfrid E. Shute. *Your Child and Vitamin E.* New Canaan, Conn.: Keats Publishing, 1979.

5
Vitamin K: The Surprise Vitamin

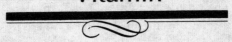

People pay little attention to vitamin K, the anti-hemorrhage vitamin, because they consider it unimportant. Actually, it is full of surprises.

First, what is vitamin K? It is a fat-soluble vitamin, the last of the group, A, D, E and K; the others, we have already discussed.

Vitamin K has an interesting history. During the years 1929 to 1933, chickens were found to be hemorrhaging if they were *fed diets low in fat*. When cabbage was given them, the chickens stopped bleeding. Since cabbage is rich in vitamin C, investigators jumped to the conclusion that the disturbance had been caused by scurvy, a vitamin C deficiency disease. The only hitch in this theory is that chickens manufacture their own vitamin C.

In 1934, H. Dam, a scientist from Copenhagen, Denmark, discovered that the hemorrhaging was due, not to a deficiency of vitamin C, but to a lack of a fat-soluble factor which, when given to the chickens, improved their coagulation ability. Dam named this factor the "Koagulation Vitamin" (as it is spelled in Denmark), and thus the name of vitamin K was born. The relationship between clotting of blood and the new vitamin was definitely established, first in animals, and, in 1937, in man.

WHERE IS VITAMIN K FOUND?

Vitamin K is found in high amounts mainly in green leafy vegetables, carrot tops and kale (in addition to the sources listed below), and in pork liver. But most important, it is found in intestinal bacteria, where it is manufactured by man.

VITAMIN K CONTENT OF RICHEST SOURCES

Sources	Dam Units per 100 grams
Putrefied fish meal	90,000
Chestnut leaves	90,000
Spinach leaves	55,000
Cabbage leaves	40,000
Cauliflower	40,000
Nettle leaves	40,000
Pine needles	20,000
Seaweed (algae)	13,000 to 17,000
Pork liver	5,000 to 10,000
Tomatoes, green	10,000
Tomatoes, ripe	5,000

Safflower, fish-liver oils and other polyunsaturated oils are also sources of vitamin K.

WHAT DOES VITAMIN K DO?

Since vitamin K is essential for blood clotting, a deficiency of this vitamin can cause hemorrhages, nosebleed and other forms of bleeding. To call K an anti-hemorrhaging vitamin is misleading; it does not necessarily stop bleeding, merely controls it. In other words, vitamin K is essential for normal blood clotting.

For example, in one study, vitamin K reduced flow in prolonged menstrual flow; clots either diminished or disappeared in many cases. In numerous cases, menstrual cramps were also lessened or abolished.

Vitamin K is needed to promote blood clotting, especially when jaundice is present.[1]

Vitamin K promotes the manufacture of thrombin (or prothrombin), the clotting factor, which takes place in the liver. However, if the liver is damaged or cannot function properly, vitamin K cannot be absorbed. If intestinal linings are damaged, the delivery of vitamin K is cut off to vital organs.

A deficiency in vitamin K can cause miscarriages.

A deficiency of vitamin K may also be a factor in sprue, diarrhea and cellular disease.

The prothrombin time (clotting time) in TB cases is restored to normal if deterioration has not progressed too far, or if there is no serious liver damage.[2]

Vitamin K has been a factor in preventing cerebral palsy. When 1 mg. of vitamin K is given to babies, immediately after birth, it has prevented it. Or, prevention has been reported if 10 to 20 mg. are given the mother during labor. (More than 10 mg. have been found toxic to infants themselves.)[3]

Vitamin K has been helpful in reducing high blood pressure in rats.[4]

Vitamin K used in 115 cancer cases showed such pain-relieving value in 73 percent of the patients that they were able to discontinue using barbiturates and morphine.[5]

Factors which interfere with vitamin K absorption are:

Frozen foods destroy vitamin K[6]

Mineral oil destroys vitamin K

Rancid fats destroy vitamin K

Prolonged use of sulfa drugs

Impaired fat assimilation

Newborn babies may need it especially

Oral antibiotics destroy vitamin K

Radiation and X rays destroy vitamin K

Chemical vapors around factories destroy vitamin K (and also vitamins A, B and C in the body)

Aspirin destroys vitamin K

Dicumarol does not destroy vitamin K, but it interferes with the action of vitamin K so the vitamin has to work twice as hard to accomplish its task

WHY ARE BILE AND FATS ABSOLUTELY NECESSARY FOR VITAMIN K ABSORPTION?

This is because it is a fat-soluble vitamin, and cannot be absorbed into the bloodstream from the intestines where it is manufactured, without fat and bile.

HOW MUCH SHOULD YOU USE?

Adelle Davis believed that if you avoid the antagonists mentioned above, and include yogurt or kefir or acidophilus in your daily diet, you may be able to manufacture a sufficient amount of your own vitamin K in your intestinal tract. Her books also recommend using unsaturated fatty acids (vegetable oils) and eating a low carbohydrate diet. These precautions increase the amount of vitamin K in the intestinal flora or bacteria, where it should flourish.[7]

Vitamin K formerly was administered in the form of concentrates of alfalfa or cereal grasses, plus the addition of bile salts for its absorption. Now vitamin K is available in tablet form. The only toxicity noted in reports occurred when large doses of synthetic vitamin K were injected into pregnant women. Usually 20 mg. per day are used orally if the need has been established. In the study of women being treated for menstrual abnormalities, 25 mg. were started just prior to menstruation and continued for five days.

The final surprise about vitamin K is that it can be used as a safe preservative to control fermentation in foods without sacrificing flavor or causing toxicity. It has no unpleasant odor, is not a pungent gas, has no bleaching effect and, when it is added to naturally colored fruits, can maintain a stable and effective condition of the foods, at the same time providing a nutrient.[8]

Apparently vitamin K is a little gem hiding its light under a bushel of ignorance.

REFERENCES

1. *Transcripts of the American Therapeutic Society.* April 9, 1954.

2. Bicknell and Prescott. *The Vitamins in Medicine.* Third Edition. Milwaukee, Wis. 53201: Lee Foundation for Nutritional Research, 1962.

3. T. C. Meyer, et al. *Archives of Diseases of Childhood.* Vol. 31, p. 212, 1956.

4. *Proceedings of the Society of Experimental Medicine and Biology.* March, 1944.

5. *Wisconsin Medical Journal.* June, 1957.

6. *Modern Nutrition.* January, 1963, p. 21.

7. Adelle Davis. *Let's Get Well.* Paperback edition. New American Library, 1972.

8. J. I. Rodale and staff. *The Complete Book of Vitamins.* Emmaus, Pa.: Rodale Books, 1966.

See also:

Ruth Adams. *Complete Home Guide to All the Vitamins.* New York: Larchmont Books, 1976.

6
The Fabulous B's

One of the earliest vitamins discovered was B, first believed a single vitamin. But, as research continued, it turned out to be a whole family of vitamins, each member related to another, yet each doing a different job. Together they comprise a "family" known as the B complex.

Most people think of the B vitamins separately, and they also take them separately. It is true that a deficiency of one may be predominant, but it is also true that, since they are always found together in nature, it is impossible to be deficient in one only. If you have signs of glaring deficiencies of one of the B vitamins, you can rest assured the deficiency of another cannot be far behind and may explode at any time. They were numbered as well as named as discovered, beginning with B-1, B-2, etc.

Complete results can only be derived from the complete complex, preferably in natural form, since here are found both the known B vitamins as well as the unknown factors not yet isolated or discovered. The researchers who were at first sure the B vitamins were only one couldn't have been more surprised when more and more began popping up. We are already up to a vitamin B-22, with still more, no doubt, coming to light in the future. So the best way to take advantage of the fabulous potentials of the B vitamin complex is to take them as a family in which all the members join hands to help you. As you discover extra need for certain members, you may add them—providing you are fortified with the entire complex to back them up. There is an important reason for this.

The American Journal of Clinical Nutrition states that in vitamin B deficiency, the administration of a single B factor may result in clinical signs of deficiency of the others.[1] Adelle Davis agreed. She wrote: "The taking of one or more of the B vitamins increases the need of the others not supplied." She gave the example of a seamstress who took more and more vitamin B-1 (thiamin) because the woman had heard that it was good for fatigue (which it is). She started out by taking it alone and felt better at first, although the effect wore off. So she tried higher and higher amounts until her hair fell out, her skin began to crack, her eyes became bloodshot and her nerves jumpy. She developed a horrendous case of eczema and became almost too tired to move. Had she taken the entire B complex, or even a small amount of thiamin together with the whole B complex, these disturbances would probably not have occurred. Yet, when I go into a drugstore, I am flabbergasted that the lowest amount of vitamin B-1 often available is not 5 or 10 mg. as it should be, but 100 mg.! I tried complaining to a few druggists, but they didn't even know what I was talking about. As Adelle Davis said, the oversupply of this or any other single B vitamin can cause deficiencies of the unsupplied vitamins that may, in turn, "produce abnormalities that can do more harm than the vitamins obtained can do good."[2]

Fatigue is not the only result of a deficiency of the B complex. We are, as a nation, becoming more and more nervous, judging by the huge amounts of tranquilizers being consumed as well as the tons of pep pills. These drugs merely cover up conditions, whereas the B complex, used as a whole, protects nerves and increases energy. The reason for the energy increase (the opposite of fatigue) is that the B complex contains essential nutrients for the endocrine glands, which regulate the machinery of the body. Vitamin B can aid in the formation of red blood cells, another energy booster. Vitamin B is definitely an antistress vitamin as well.

What are the symptoms of too little vitamin B?

If you are tired, irritable, nervous, feel frightened, depressed or even suicidal, suspect a B deficiency. If you have gray hair, falling hair, baldness, acne or other skin troubles, suspect a lack of vitamin B. If you suffer from poor appetite, insomnia, neuritis, anemia, constipation or high cholesterol, you may need vitamin B. If your tongue is enlarged (including the buds at each side) and is shiny, bright red and full of grooves, you definitely need B.

Bicknell and Prescott, in their technical reference book, *The Vitamins in Medicine,* published in England, state that cases of senile dementia in mental hospitals and convalescent homes have exhibited a dramatic improvement in their mental condition in twenty-four to forty-eight hours after large doses of the B vitamins.[3] Mental hospitals using B vitamins have found them more successful than drugs. One person testified that the therapy of Dr. Miles Atkinson, which consisted of heavy intakes of vitamin B four times daily, reversed his severe condition of Ménière's disease, which had lasted almost four months. The B vitamin treatment relieved within two months the dizziness, double vision, nausea and inability to concentrate and saved the man's sanity, as well as his job. Heart abnormalities have also responded to the use of the B complex; the nerves affecting the heart need vitamin B for smooth, quiet function.

The list could go on and on. More symptoms will be discussed as we examine the individual B vitamins in subsequent chapters. And most people will recognize one or more symptoms of the deficiency of vitamin B in themselves. One reason there is so much B vitamin deficiency in the American population is because we eat so many processed foods from which the B's have often been removed. If you eat enriched flour or cereals, this does not solve the problem because, as I have said earlier, up to twenty-three natural nutrients have often been removed and three synthetics have been substituted. Another reason for widespread deficiency is the high amount of sugar Americans eat. Sugar, and alcohol, gobble up vitamin B, leaving the poor host defenseless. But there is another pitfall. The B vitamins are water-soluble, instead of fat-soluble as are vitamins A, D, E and K. This means they are dissolved in water (or liquids), cannot be stored in the body, but must be continuously replaced. Alcohol is one of the greatest known causes of both using up and washing the B vitamins out of the body. During World War II, even the Navy discovered that taking B vitamins with cocktails could prevent a hangover. And other liquids, including too much coffee, have been found to wash away B vitamins, sometimes resulting in gray hair.

I am sure by this time you are wondering where you can get B complex to hopefully correct the many symptoms mentioned, or prevent them from developing. The

B complex is the hardest to get in supplement form because capsules do not hold enough, or at least not as much as the foods that supply these valuable nutrients. Adelle Davis said: "Let us be cautious in feeling secure that a mere capsule of mixed B vitamins will supply the body's requirements . . . our needs must be met largely by wholesome foods chosen with the utmost care."[4]

The foods rich in vitamin B are liver, brewer's yeast, wheat germ, rice polish and blackstrap molasses. Brewer's yeast contains a minimum of ten B vitamins (and probably many more) and has been credited with almost miraculous recovery from deficiency states ranging from skin disturbances to lack of energy within hours, days or a few weeks. (Calcium should always be added when taking brewer's yeast, as I will explain in a later chapter.) Fortunately, if conditions are ideal, you can manufacture some of your own B vitamins in your intestinal tract. But conditions are not always ideal. If you are on a fat-free diet or if you have taken antibiotics, your manufacture may cease. The intestinal bacteria or flora must be in an A-1 state. Unsaturated fats, particularly linoleic acid, stimulate the growth of the friendly intestinal flora while antibiotics kill them. This explains why most European doctors, and many in America, prescribe substances to fortify and re-build the flora when they prescribe antibiotics.

Yogurt, buttermilk, kefir, acidophilus or bifidus taken during or after a course of antibiotics, will usually do the job. If, when you take brewer's yeast ranging from a teaspoon a day upward in juices, you suffer from gas, it is a usual sign that you are either deficient in the friendly intestinal flora or hydrochloric acid, both of which are often needed for its digestion.

How much vitamin B do you need? Who knows? How big are you? The bigger your frame, the more cells you own and the more cells, the greater the need for vitamin B to nourish those cells. How much sugar do you eat? How much alcohol do you drink? How much processed food do you eat? How many of the vitamin B-rich foods do you eat? You will have to analyze your own needs.

Remember that vitamin B complex capsules are not to be shunned. Even Adelle Davis admitted to taking six daily, but this is not enough. The B complex foods are necessary, too. And don't forget those B complex capsules should be in natural form—the source of *all,* not a few, B vitamins. As Adelle Davis said, she has never seen gray hair resume its natural color on synthetic B vitamins, but she has noted this phenomenon, if it happens at all, after the person has eaten plenty of B vitamin complex *whole* foods.

Following is the list of the separate B vitamins so far discovered. Become familiar with them. We will discuss most of them in the next chapters, which provide some exciting information. A few are so new that nobody knows what they accomplish.

Vitamin B-1 (also known as thiamin or thiamin chloride), B-2 (riboflavin), B-3 (niacin, nicotinic acid, niacinamide and nicotinamide), B-6 (pyridoxine), B-12, B-13, B-14, B-15, B-17, B-22, choline, inositol, folic acid, pantothenic acid, para-amino-benzoic acid (usually called PABA), biotin and orotic acid have been already identified.

As I have said, we will discuss the B vitamins one by one, but before we begin, have a look at your tongue. According to Adelle Davis, it is the telltale sign of deficiencies of the individual B vitamins.

TONGUE SYMPTOM INDICATES VITAMIN B FACTOR LACK
A scarred tongue . . . . Vitamin B-1 (thiamin)
deficiency

A purplish or magenta tongue	Vitamin B-2 (riboflavin) deficiency
A fiery red tongue tip, too..... small or too large tongue, a coating of fuzzy debris	Vitamin B-3 (niacin) deficiency (The fuzzy debris shows putrefaction in the intestines.)
A beefy tongue...............	Panthothenic acid deficiency.
A smooth, beefy strawberry red tongue (the smoothness being noticeable at the tip and sides)	Vitamin B-12 and folic acid deficiencies.

In a severe overall vitamin B deficiency there are fissures and cracks in the tongue which resemble the relief map of the Grand Canyon.

Actually, there is probably no such thing as a deficiency of a single B vitamin factor. The factors are too closely related. Like members of the family, one helps another. Good results happen faster when brewer's yeast or liver (in desiccated tablet form if you don't like the food) or both, are used to knit the whole tribe together (and taken on the same day) you may be taking a single B vitamin in addition. These foods are the richest sources of *all* the B vitamins, and they not only help you feel better faster, but give you much value for your money.

Now let's look to see what vitamins B-1 and B-2 can do to help you.

REFERENCES

1. *The American Journal of Clinical Nutrition.* November, 1962, p. 334.

2. Adelle Davis. *Let's Eat Right to Keep Fit.* Paperback edition. New York: New American Library, 1970.

3. Bicknell and Prescott. *The Vitamins in Medicine.* Third Edition. Milwaukee, Wis. 53201: Lee Foundation for Nutritional Research, 1962.

4. Adelle Davis, *op. cit.*

See also:

Ruth Adams and Frank Murray. *Body, Mind and the B Vitamins.* New York: Larchmont Books, 1972.

Abram Hoffer and Morton Walker. *Nutrients to Age Without Senility.* New Canaan, Conn.: Keats Publishing, 1980.

7
Vitamins B-1 and B-2

It was 1867 and Dr. Christian Eijkmann had been sent by the Dutch government to the Island of Java to try to find the cause of a strange disease among the Javanese prisoners. The men were staggering and no one understood why. Medical treatment had failed. Dr. Eijkmann nearly failed, too, until chickens in the prison barnyard exhibited the same symptoms as the prisoners.

When he investigated, he found that there was a connection: the chickens were being fed the leftovers from the prisoners' plates, a diet that consisted mostly of boiled white rice, the chief fare of the prisoners. The doctor tried adding the rice polishings, which had been removed from the white rice, to the diet, and both prisoners and chickens recovered.

The coating on rice contains vitamin B-1, which helps to digest the starchy content of the rice. Ordinarily, this coating is removed from natural brown rice and sold back as a vitamin supplement today, at double the price, to people who eat white rice. What folly, when we could all eat brown rice in the first place. The flavor, as well as the nutritive value, is far superior to that of white rice, and we would be protected against the strange disease of the Javanese prisoners and chickens, which was named beri beri.

VITAMIN B-1 (THIAMIN)

B-1, or thiamin, is still used today for beri-beri. Few doctors are aware of this disease and often prescribe drugs for its symptoms instead of realizing that it is a deficiency disease due to the lack of thiamin. To show you how effective this vitamin can be, in a recent hospital study of beri-beri adult cases,[1] thiamin produced the following improvements:

Diuresis (excretion of excess fluid stored in the body) within twenty-four to forty-eight hours

Decrease in rapid heart rate

Reduction of enlarged heart (It has been known to reduce an enlarged heart in a matter of weeks, or less.)

Normalization of electrocardiogram

Clearing of pulmonary congestion

Since 1867, vitamin B-1 (or thiamin chloride or thiamin) has been found to have a finger in many other pies. According to numerous studies it can also aid in:

Manufacture of hydrochloric acid

Protection against ulcers

Brain nourishment

Restoring appetite and improving food assimilation and digestion, particularly of starches, sugars and alcohol (As I said in the preceding chapter, the Navy officers of World War II discovered it was an excellent preventive for hangovers.)

Eliminating nausea

Calming nerves and preventing nervous breakdowns

Reversing lethargy, loss of morale as well as loss of sense of humor

Improving muscle tone

Improving circulation

Preventing fatigue and increasing stamina

Building blood

Relieving constipation

Improving an abnormally low thyroid

Relieving irritability

Eliminating edema (fluid retention) in connection with degenerative heart conditions

Eliminating neuritis

Overcoming sciatica, that excruciating pain running down the sciatic nerve from hip to ankle

Protecting nerves against too loud noises; a help for insomnia

If you have any such symptoms, you may need more thiamin (B-1). These symptoms may also be due to other causes, but if you have several of them, a deficiency of B-1 may be the culprit.

WHAT FOODS CONTAIN VITAMIN B-1 IN ABUNDANCE?

Brewer's yeast is the richest source of this vitamin. Next, in descending order, are the germs of grains—wheat germ and barley germ; then the wholegrains themselves—wholewheat, oatmeal, whole brown rice (or the rice polishings themselves); nuts and nut butters; and finally, meats, particularly kidney, heart and pork. Soybeans are high in B-1, too.

Cooking and the use of soda in cooking destroys B-1. The worst practice of all is to flood vegetables, which contain some B vitamins, with water, overcook them and then pour the water down the sink. Remember, all B vitamins are water-soluble, meaning that they dissolve in water.

If you use too much water in cooking and then throw the cooking water down the sink, you are nourishing the sink, not you. Save this water for soups, juices, etc.

HOW MUCH B-1 SHOULD YOU TAKE?

B-1, of course, also comes in supplement form. I refuse to speculate how much you should take. I do know it is disturbing to take too much of it without the other members of the B complex. You may want to reread here the story in the preceding chapter about the seamstress who took too much B-1. A small amount of thiamin made the seamstress feel better, but the effect soon wore off and she had to increase the dose. This, in turn, also wore off. As she took larger and larger doses, she became worse and worse. Some of her symptoms were those of a B-1 deficiency; but as she progressed, other symptoms developed, indicating deficiencies of the other B vitamins, too, showing that too much of one can create an imbalance and deficiency of the others. Adelle Davis said: "Large doses of B-1 alone can cause a high urinary excretion of other B vitamins so that deficiencies of the other B vitamins can be produced."[2]

It is true that a doctor may give a patient an emergency injection of a massive amount of B-1, but he does not continue this indefinitely.

VITAMIN B-2 (RIBOFLAVIN)

Vitamin B-2, or riboflavin, has not received as much attention as vitamin B-1. This may be because it has not been studied as thoroughly, or perhaps because it is "newer" than B-1. Of course, all of these vitamins have always been where nature put them: in natural foods. They are merely new to those researchers who have discovered them and their health values. Nevertheless, vitamin B-2 has a great many successes attributed to it.

The most common symptoms of a lack of B-2 are the following conditions:

Cracks and sores in the corners of the mouth and a red and sore tongue

A feeling of grit or sand on the inside of the eyelids, also, burning of the eyes, and being disturbed by very bright light

Scaling around the nose and mouth, forehead and ears

Trembling, sluggishness, dizziness and a certain type of abnormal sensation in the legs

Anemia (There are other causes of anemia, but a B-2 deficiency can be a factor.)

Dropsy

Inability to urinate

Vaginal itching

Diabetes (B-2 may be only one factor.)

Ulcers

Eczema

Baldness

Gummed eyelids

Conjunctivitis

Oily skin, whiteheads and oily hair

Experimental studies show that some forms of cancer may be related to a B-2 deficiency, and certainly the lack of this vitamin has been a factor in birth defects. The tragic deformities from the use of thalidomide were traced to the door of a B-2 deficiency. Had the pregnant mother had enough of this vitamin in her diet, researchers state, the baby might have been protected from the hideous abnormalities.

The most recent and exciting finding about B-2 is its role in helping to prevent some types of cataracts. The most electrifying discovery was that concentrated galactose (a form of milk sugar) is an antagonist to B-2, creating a deficiency of the vitamin in the body that can lead, in some cases, to the formation of at least one type of cataract.[3] (There are, as I have noted, various causes of cataracts.)

Researchers have learned that a lack of B-2 can cause cataracts in both animals and humans. Dr. P. S. Day of Columbia University and Dr. Lewis Sydenstricker at the University of Georgia, learned that this vitamin could also reverse cataracts if it were given long enough and in high enough doses. Forty-seven patients at the University of Georgia were suffering from eye ailments; six had fully developed cataracts. When the patients were given 15 mg. of B-2 daily, various eye symptoms improved within twenty-four hours, though some patients needed an additional twenty-four hours for results. The eye disturbances that responded quickly were: general eye weakness, poor vision, sensitivity to light, burning and itching eyelids. Cataracts required nine months of therapeutic doses (15 mg. daily) to be reabsorbed. As a conclusive test, some of these patients were deprived of the B-2. Their cataract symptoms returned, but when the B-2 treatment was resumed, the cataracts were again reversed.[4] (Remember, however, that insufficient B-2 is not the only culprit in cataracts.[5])

It is difficult to get sufficient riboflavin from foods. The richest source is brewer's yeast, though liver, kidney and heart, as well as soybeans and flour, wholewheat products, hickory nuts, hazel nuts and peanuts, contain a fair amount.

Most of the single B vitamins are synthetic. If there is a great need for one or more of these vitamins, the synthetic form may be necessary for a short while, or, if needed in a serious condition (as in cataracts), for a longer period.[5] If one were to take these vitamins, particularly B-2, in natural food form, it would undoubtedly take much, much longer to accomplish results, since more foods contain so little. So it is wise to take both B-2 supplements and B complex foods.

REFERENCES

1. *American Journal of Clinical Nutrition.* August, 1970, p. 1017.

2. Adelle Davis. *Let's Get Well.* Paperback edition. New York: New American Library, 1972.

3. *The Archives of Opthalmology.* Vol. 65, p. 181, 1967.

4. *Ibid.*

5. Linda Clark. *Handbook of Natural Remedies for Common Ailments.* Old Greenwich, Conn.: Devin Adair Company, 1976.

See also:

Joyce Hoffman and the editors of *Prevention* magazine. *Here's to Your Health.* Emmaus, Pa.: Rodale Press, 1980.

8
Vitamin B-3:
A Wonder Worker

Vitamin B-3, niacin, is a dramatic vitamin, accomplishing miracles such as no other vitamin can boast. It is known as the vitamin used to treat the three D's: dermatitis, diarrhea and dementia. Although chemists discovered it more than seventy-five years ago, no one seemed to know at the time its value or that it was a member of the vitamin B family. The route by which these discoveries were finally made is almost laughable, though at the time, it was far from being a laughing matter.

At the turn of the century, pellagra was a worldwide problem. It was especially prevalent in our Southern states, where approximately 100,000 cases a year were followed by 10,000 deaths. No cause or cure had been found. Some doctors were convinced that it was caused by a germ or a mold. Other doctors were sure it was caused by a gnat, found on buffalo. For twenty-three years the search for a clue continued. Finally, Dr. Joseph Goldberger isolated the cause and announced to a red-faced medical association that pellagra was actually a vitamin deficiency disease and the missing vitamin was niacin, a vitamin that had been lost in the refining process in degerminating cornmeal, a staple of the Southern diet.

Today the cornmeal situation is not much improved. Try and find cornmeal that has not been degerminated in any supermarket! Undegerminated cornmeal, however, is available in health stores. Thus, as in the case of the missing rice polishings containing thiamin (B-1) that resulted in the deficiency disease, beri-beri (discussed in the preceding chapter), a second deficiency disease was now proved by Dr. Goldberger to be caused by the folly of man trying to outsmart nature.

The amazing thing about niacin is the speed with which it can reverse disorders. For example, Adelle Davis wrote: "I have known of dozens of persons, many of whom have had diarrhea for years, whose problem cleared up in a day or two after natural sources of B vitamins and 100 mg. of niacinamide were taken with each meal."[1]

What else can niacin accomplish? It has had positive effects on the following disturbances:

Atherosclerosis (hardening or a clogging up of the arteries), vertigo, and some cases of progressive deafness that have been halted or slightly improved.[2]

It has been found helpful for elderly patients who are mentally confused.[3]

Doctors often use it as one method to increase circulation to cramping, painful legs in the elderly, although there are other methods of relief for this problem, too.

Lack of niacin has been found to cause malformations in baby mice. In fact, a temporary interference of niacin synthesis in the mothers' bodies was discovered to be a factor in malformed children after the mothers had been given thalidomide.[4]

A deficiency of niacin can lead to loss of memory,

bad breath, small ulcers, canker sores, dizziness, insomnia, irritability, nausea, vomiting, recurring headaches, sensations of strain, tension and deep depression. Niacin is also known to be essential to provide hydrochloric acid for impaired digestion.

Niacin has been found to improve six out of seven patients with neurasthenia. It also has increased responsiveness and improved sleep and has been used for schizophrenia.[5]

But you should also know about a peculiarity of the vitamin.

One function of niacin is similar to that of thiamin (B-1): both help burn starch and sugar in the body. Another function of niacin is to stimulate peripheral circulation, one that can create possible panic for the uninitiated. Niacin was formerly called nicotinic acid. They are the same vitamin. When taken in food, it does not cause any problems, but when taken in tablet form, it has a surprising—though temporary—effect that may scare you out of your wits if you don't expect it. In most people, about fifteen minutes after taking a niacin tablet, it causes an intense flush. You may turn beet red, burn like crazy, prickle and itch. Sometimes it is more noticeable in some parts of your body than others; it may be your head, face, feet, legs, arms, or all over. This effect merely means that your circulation has really been stirred up in various parts of your body. The flush is not considered dangerous, rather an anti-histamine factor. It lasts for approximately fifteen minutes, then it is all over.

There are two synthetic forms of niacin that have had the flushing property removed. They are called niacinamide and nicotinamide. But some disturbances may not respond to these forms as they do to niacin or nicotinic acid. One of these disturbances is acne; the other, that old bogey, migraine headache.

An English doctor discovered by chance that niacin was successful in all of the twenty cases of acne he treated. He said: "The patients who develop facial flush do better with this treatment." His initial dose was 100 mg. three times daily, continued for two to three weeks or until regular flushing was experienced.[6]

Lewis J. Silvers, M.D., writes: "Many a migraine headache can be prevented from developing into the excruciatingly painful stage by taking niacin at the first sign of an attack. Migraine usually gives ample warning: spots appear to obstruct vision and flashes of light further complicate the picture; nausea comes early, and is later followed by headache and vomiting. At the very first symptoms, even if they wake you out of a sound sleep, immediately take 50 mg. of niacin. If a flush ensues, the dose is sufficient to quickly dilate the constricted cerebral blood vessels. If you do not flush, take another tablet, so that you *will* flush. Presto, no migraine."[7]

Miles Atkinson, M.D., an otologist, now retired from the faculty of New York University, has used niacin for both migraine and Ménière's disease (vertigo) as well as for associated cases of deafness and tinnitus. Dr. Atkinson wisely added other factors to the patient's diet, too: B-1, B-2, B-6, calcium pantothenate (another B vitamin), as well as ascorbic acid (vitamin C) and desiccated liver. The results were helpful for many.[8]

The miracles wrought by niacin by no means stop here. Drs. Richard M. Halpern and Roberts A. Smith, of the Molecular Biology Institute, report research that the flushless nicotinamide may be a factor in preventing cancer, due to enzyme regulation that apparently protects normal cells and prevents them from becoming malignant. Their studies revealed that malignancy was, in some way, associated with a deficiency of niacin. To prove that it could help prevent cancer, they exposed isolated malignant cells in their laboratory to nicotinamide and watched the vitamin suppress further malignancy. The doctors admit they do not know the dosage that should be used for this purpose, since individual needs vary.[9]

Some people who have taken niacin and have not experienced the flush wonder why. One explanation is that if a flush is not forthcoming, it is connected with the anti-histamine factor. Some physicians suspect that the liver is not functioning properly; in fact, this is often used as a test of liver dysfunction. It is also true that after continuous dosage of niacin for an indefinite time, the flush stops.

Foods rich in niacin include whole grains, rice bran, rice polishings, nuts and roasted peanuts, poultry, liver and yeast. One tablespoon of brewer's yeast (if small flakes) or two tablespoons (if large flakes) contain 10 mg. niacin, or approximately one ounce. You will recall that Dr. Goldberger returned his patients to health on *brewer's yeast (three ounces daily)*. This food, which also contains the other B vitamins, minerals and protein, is easy to stir into a drink of juice or even water. It is also an excellent energy pickup. One slice of liver contains 16.1 mg. of niacin, plus many other factors. Ten 10-grain tablets of desiccated liver equal one ounce of fresh liver.

As for toxicity of the niacin tablets, E. Cheraskin, M.D., D.M.D., and W. M. Ringsdorf Jr., D.M.D., M.S., report that neither niacin, nicotinic acid nor the amides are toxic. They consider them safer than aspirin. However, they do believe that, taken in tablet form, niacin may cause headache and nausea in some cases. They believe that niacin in foods is a better choice for chronic cases.[10] (There is usually no flush from niacin foods or from the supplement niacinamide).

But there is another side to the story of nontoxicity. Large doses of niacin or nicotinic acid have been found to reduce cholesterol,[11] but in my research, I keep coming across warnings against taking too much niacin (in tablets, not foods). Later warnings have cited cases of jaundice resulting from using large amounts of the vitamin for cholesterol-lowering purposes.[12,13] *The American Journal of Clinical Nutrition* has also warned of the danger.[14] Adelle Davis wrote: "Massive doses of niacin given to reduce blood cholesterol for more than a year have developed stomach ulcers, severe liver damage, diabetes, jaundice and colitis; men have reported sexual impotence.[15]

Whether the disturbing results are due to creating an imbalance of the other vitamins by taking large amounts of one has not been proved, to my knowledge, except in the cases of B-1, B-2 and B-6.

You have, of course, heard of megavitamin therapy. Mega means "great," so megavitamin denotes great amounts of a vitamin. Great amounts of niacin have been used with success for treating schizophrenia. The psychiatrists who use this massive dose therapy do not believe that it causes an imbalance of the other B vitamins. They feel, rather, that in schizophrenia, there is already a mental deficiency or imbalance; and for the mentally ill, the vitamin in large amounts can help to establish balance. This seems to be a different story from a high dosage for the normal person who is not mentally ill. The two psychiatrists, Dr. Abram Hoffer and Dr. Humphry Osmond, who initiated this therapy have found no serious toxicity from niacin or its other forms in mentally disturbed or schizophrenic patients, even when used as long as ten to fifteen years. So this may be why reports of the use of niacin for normal people and for schizophrenics conflict.[16]

REFERENCES

1. Adelle Davis. *Let's Get Well.* Paperback edition. New York: New American Library, 1972.

2. *Nutritional Abstracts and Reviews.* July, 1962. Abstract No. 4257.

3. Abram Hoffer and Morton Walker. *Nutrients to Age Without Senility.* New Canaan, Connecticut: Keats Publishing, Inc., 1980.

4. *Nutritional Abstracts and Reviews.* January, 1967. Abstract No. 431.

5. *Nutritional Abstracts and Reviews.* July, 1962. Abstract No. 4257.

6. *British Medical Journal.* December 16, 1967.

7. Lewis J. Silvers. *Doctor Silvers' Extraordinary Remedies for Health and Longevity.* Englewood Cliffs, N.J.: Prentice-Hall, 1964.

8. *Archives of Otolaryngology.* Vol. 75, p. 220. 1962.

9. Richard M. Halpern and Roberts A. Smith. *Organic Consumer Report.* July 27, 1971.

10. E. Cheraskin and W. M. Ringsdorf, Jr. *New Hope for Incurable Disease.* Paperback edition. New York: Arco Publishing, 1973.

11. *Nutritional Abstracts and Reviews.* April, 1968. Abstract No. 2503.

12. *Nutritional Abstracts and Reviews.* April, 1962. Abstract Nos. 2582 and 2583.

13. *Nutritional Abstracts and Reviews.* October, 1962. Abstract No. 5309.

14. *American Journal of Clinical Nutrition.* July-August, 1960, p. 478.

15. Adelle Davis, *op. cit.*

16. Abram Hoffer and Humphry Osmond. *How to Live with Schizophrenia.* Paperback edition. Secaucus, N.J.: Citadel Press (Lyle Stuart), 1978.

See also:

Carlton Fredericks. *Psycho-Nutrition.* New York: Grosset & Dunlap, 1976.

William H. Philpott and Dwight K. Kalita. *Brain Allergies.* New Canaan, Conn.: Keats Publishing, 1980.

9
Vitamin B-6: Pyridoxine

Have you ever wondered if there were a vitamin that could help you reduce? Or one to stop those excruciating charley horses in the calves of your legs in the middle of the night? Or one that could help certain types of painful arthritic hands? Or even one that could bring a little welcome relief to women prior to their menstrual periods or during menopause? Well, there is one. It is vitamin B-6 (pyridoxine). But before you jump out of your chair to go buy some at the nearest health store, learn the whole story.

Vitamin B-6 may indeed help with an overweight problem, providing it is caused by the water storage problem in the body known as edema. John M. Ellis, M.D. of Texas, who devoted many years of study of the effects of B-6 on his thousands of patients, found that this vitamin sets up a balance of the minerals sodium and potassium in the body. These minerals in turn regulate the body fluids and help eliminate the edema without the use of a diuretic drug, which so often creates serious side effects. Dr. Ellis found that both men and women were helped by B-6.

Cattlemen who ride the vast Texas range reported to Dr. Ellis that after using B-6 as he directed, tingling and numbness in their fingers and toes—as well as the night cramps in the calves of their legs—ceased. Even more surprising, without diuretics or a change in diet, these men found that they could tighten their belts to the last notch, due to the loss of excess fluid from their bodies.

Many women are said to become witches during their premenstrual periods. Abdomens bloat, breasts swell, weight increases due to water storage. This condition is called premenstrual edema. B-6 can help by preventing a buildup of water in the tissues. Emotional problems also flare at this time, partially because of a drop in blood sugar and calcium. This can be alleviated by eating often (protein foods, not sweets), avoiding too much coffee (which disturbs the blood sugar level) and supplying more calcium. Otherwise, a normally pleasant woman may have a personality change. She can become quarrelsome, irritable and depressed; she can indeed be hard to live with.

Adelle Davis quoted one woman as saying: "This is the time I spank the kids, yell at my husband, live on tranquilizers and can't stand myself."[1] Dr. Erle Henricksen of the University of California adds: "It takes extremely stable husbands and children to put up with the worst sufferers."[2] By controlling the blood sugar syndrome, using vitamin E routinely throughout the month, adding calcium and B-6, it has been possible to prevent these temporary premenstrual changes.

Dr. Ellis found that B-6 was extremely successful for women who suffered from premenstrual edema. He also found that women, and even men, who neared the age of menopause often developed painful spurs or knots on the sides of their finger joints. These appendages were accompanied by painful arm and shoulder symptoms. But after the administration of B-6, there was a dramatic change. Finger joints ceased to be painful within about six weeks. Within two weeks, there was often a loss of as much as five to seven pounds. Wedding rings could once more be slipped off fingers that had become fat and puffy. Women could use thimbles, thread needles more easily and dropped fewer dishes. In other words, the B-6 improved finger sensitivity and hand flexion. All of this is told in the fascinating book *The Doctor Who Looked at Hands* by Dr. Ellis. It is the story of his exciting research with B-6.[3]

What else can B-6 accomplish? Dr. Douw G. Stern of the University of South Africa discovered that Parkinson's disease, a nervous disorder that causes trembling or hand-shakiness, responds to B-6. He cites a case of Parkinsonism that had existed for twenty-five years but responded to B-6 injections within two months. (Magnesium, a co-worker with B-6, may hasten improvement with this malady.) This is one of the unexpected results of B-6: whereas it may take a long time to derive benefits from some vitamins, B-6 seems to work quickly and sometimes dramatically.

Dr. Miriam Benner reported that by giving a massive dose (under medical supervision) of 2,000 mg. of B-6 daily, a woman who had been paralyzed on the left side of her body as a result of an operation was helped even though the treatment started two and one-half years after the operation. Dr. Benner stated: "It (B-6) produced fantastic, unexpected improvement."[4]

Many people know that B-6 can help prevent nausea in pregnancy, but they may not know it has also been used to prevent both edema and toxemia in pregnancy.

Mothers who took B-6 during pregnancy seemed to produce children who were healthier, both mentally and physically, according to Dr. Ellis. He prescribed high doses of B-6 to pregnant woman (usually 50 mg. twice daily). To others, he gave 50 mg. daily, and rarely prescribed more, although in some difficult cases he raised the dosage to 100 mg. daily. He does not believe that the Recommended Dietary Allowance of B-6 is sufficient to accomplish the full B-6 potential. He prescribed 50 mg. daily to patients who took it as long as three years without displaying any side effects.[5] Today some people take even more without side effects.

Other research has confirmed the value of B-6. The U.S. Medical Research and Nutritional Laboratory at Fitzsimmons General Hospital in Denver has found that vitamin B-6 seems to be a protection in epilepsy as well as in abnormal brain function. When B-6 was removed from the diet of one healthy young man, he developed grand mal (epileptic convulsions).[6] So far, these researchers believe that B-6 does not cure epilepsy but can prevent or lessen seizures.

What else can B-6 accomplish? The list is legion. It has helped:

One form of anemia[7]
Male sexual disorders
Eczema
Thinning and loss of hair
Elevated cholesterol
Diarrhea (Pantothenic acid and magnesium may also be needed.)
Hemorrhoids (Adelle Davis reported a "miraculous recovery" following the use of 10 mg. of B-6 after each meal.)[8]

Some types of visual disturbances

Pancreatitis

Insomnia (Pantothenic acid, magnesium and calcium can be added.)

Ulcers

Muscular weakness (One-half of the body's store of B-6 is concentrated in muscles.)

Some types of heart disturbances (The heart is a muscle and also needs B-6.)

Burning feet

Some types of kidney stones, especially when the body overproduces oxalic acid that may lead to the formation of such stones (Adequate magnesium and B-6 have slowed down this overproduction of oxalic acid in the bodies of those afflicted.)

Diabetes and low blood sugar, with which B-6 seems to be associated

Infections (B-6 seems to act as a natural antihistamine, a lack of which prevents the manufacture of antibodies that fight infection.)

The peripheral nerves (One of the greatest advantages of B-6 seems to be its ability to eliminate numbness and tingling of the toes and fingers, that "going to sleep" feeling in the extremities.)

It is required for the absorption of vitamin B-12

It is required for the production of hydrochloric acid

It is an aid in acne

It has been found to prevent tooth decay[9]

It is an important source of energy

There are certain antagonists, or special properties of B-6 about which you should know.

1. Army researchers found that the greater amount

of protein in the diet, the greater the need for B-6 to help metabolize the protein.[10] The solution is not to cut down on protein, but to step up B-6 according to Dr. Ellis.

2. Fasting can deplete the body's store of B-6.

3. A reducing diet can interfere with the body's supply of B-6. Carbohydrates also need B-6 to assist their metabolism.

4. The University of Taiwan discovered that the more exercise one takes, the more B-6 one needs.

5. Some drugs (including "The Pill") can interfere with B-6.

6. According to the University of Delaware, B-6 is involved in the metabolism of essential fatty acids.

7. B-6 is destroyed by sunlight, oxidation and heat. Cooking at 245°F. destroys vitamin B-6. Food processing and refining destroy or eliminate it.

8. B-6 seems to be another B vitamin that, if given alone, can cause an imbalance or deficiency of other B vitamins. As an example, the Army study found that by boosting the intake of B-6, a secondary deficiency of B-3 or niacin was created.[11] B-6 supplements, also known as pyridoxine, are synthetic. For protection from imbalance when taking supplements of B-6, always add some natural food that contains all the B vitamins.[12] As a matter of fact, three tablespoons of brewer's yeast will supply your daily quota of B-6 as well as the other B vitamins.

Raw foods contain more B-6 than cooked foods, since cooking and processing remove or destroy B-6. Raw foods especially rich in B-6 are bananas, avocados, green leafy vegetables, green peppers, cabbage, carrots and peanuts. Brewer's yeast and wheat germ can also be eaten raw. Pecans are an especially rich source. Dr. Ellis found that by giving his patients twelve raw pecans daily a form of painful shoulder, arm and hand neuritis disappeared within six weeks.

REFERENCES

1. Adelle Davis. *Let's Get Well.* Paperback edition. New York: New American Library, 1972.

2. Linda Clark. *Stay Young Longer.* Paperback edition. New York: Pyramid Communications, 1968.

3. John M. Ellis. *The Doctor Who Looked at Hands.* Paperback edition. New York: Arco Publishing, 1970. See also: John M. Ellis, M.D. and James Presley. *The Doctor's Report.* New York: Harper and Row, 1973.

4. *Journal of the American Medical Women's Association.* November, 1964.

5. John M. Ellis, *op. cit.*

6. J. I. Rodale and staff. *The Complete Book of Vitamins.* Emmaus, Pa.: Rodale Books, 1966.

7. Carl C. Pfeiffer. *Mental and Elemental Nutrients.* New Canaan, Conn.: Keats Publishing, Inc., 1975.

8. Adelle Davis, *op. cit.*

9. *New York State Dental Journal.* March, 1958.

10. *Annals of the New York Academy of Sciences.* Vol. 166, p. 16, 1969.

Also: Science News Letter. November 30, 1968.

11. *Annals of the New York Academy of Sciences, op. cit.*

12. *Ibid.*

10
Vitamin B-12 and Folic Acid

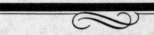

In 1948, a woman was bedfast, suffering from an upset stomach, a sore mouth, a shortness of breath and overwhelming fatigue. Her face exhibited a ghastly pallor. She was a victim of pernicious anemia, a disease due to failure of the body to manufacture enough red blood cells in the bone marrow. Whereas her red blood count should have been 4.5 million (red blood corpuscles per cubic millimeter), it was only 1.5 million, considered a seriously low level. Prior to 1948, the verdict for such patients would have been death. But due to a then-recent discovery, this woman won a reprieve, and with her, many other victims of pernicious anemia all over the world.

Thanks to the unrelenting search for an antipernicious anemia factor, not only was a specific help found for this dread disease, but a new vitamin was born. Dr. Randolph West, of New York City's Presbyterian Hospital, in collaboration with Merck Laboratories, isolated, from many tons of liver, a few, tiny red needlelike crystals. When five-millionths of an ounce of this newly found substance was injected into the muscle of the previously doomed woman, a dramatic change occurred. Six weeks after the injection, her blood count had become normal and she was in good health. The substance responsible was christened vitamin B-12.

Since 1948, other ailments have been found to respond to vitamin B-12, many with dramatic effects, according to researchers. These ailments include neuritis resulting from diabetes mellitus and chronic alcoholism; osteoarthritis and osteoporosis; multiple sclerosis and spastic paraplegia; cerebellar atrophy and polyneuritis. Even bursitis and asthma have yielded to vitamin B-12 therapy.

A B-12 deficiency can be a factor in tobacco blindness, known as amblyopia, and sufficient B-12 has been found to prevent it.[1] The blindness is due to large amounts of cyanide in tobacco. The cyanide causes the degeneration of the myelin sheath, a covering that protects the nerves. The optic nerve is the first nerve to be affected by the poison. Fortunately, if enough B-12 is given early enough to prevent the nerve deterioration, complete recovery is possible. Don't forget that tobacco poisoning is not limited to smokers. For those who are constantly subjected to the smoking of others, tobacco can also be a hazard. So, in addition to its use for pernicious anemia, B-12 is also considered "a nerve vitamin." Stress increases the need for B-12 too. But there is still more help available from B-12.

In addition to the hazards of a vitamin B-12 deficiency already mentioned, Oded Abramsky, M.D., of the Neurology Department of Hadassah University in Jerusalem, cites the following changes in the nervous system that may occur: soreness and weakness in legs and arms; diminished reflex response and sensory perception; difficulty in walking and speaking (stammering) and jerking of limbs. These symptoms may not be noted until permanent mental deterioration and paralysis occur. If caught in time by medical diagnosis, B-12 can help.

Lack of B-12 has also been found to cause a type of brain damage, resembling schizophrenia. Actually, the mental symptoms differ; they may not be consistent at all, but may express themselves in difficulty of concentration, agitation or moodiness, to maniacal behavior, even hallucinations. In physical diagnosis, the cause of this type of brain damage may elude a doctor who is looking for the usual nervous symptoms of B-12 deficiency—sore mouth, numbness or stiffness, a feeling of deadness or shooting pains, needles-and-pins or hot-and-cold sensations. Actually, the symptoms of the B-12 type of brain damage— that can range from depression and loss of mental energy to full-fledged psychosis—have been found to be a pre-pernicious anemia state. Even nutritional doctors can be caught unaware because some of these symptoms are similar to those indicating deficiencies of B-6 and magnesium. This is why, in nutritional therapy or prevention of illness, separate nutrients should not be relied upon as a panacea. *All nutrients are needed.* Vitamins and minerals work as a team for best results, either for prevention or for treatment.[2] And, as you will soon see, in the case of vitamin B-12, prevention is much easier than cure for a deficiency of the vitamin. Once serious manifestations of its lack have occurred, it is not a do-it-yourself treatment.

B-12 is not only difficult to get in food, it is difficult to assimilate by mouth. This is why, in serious conditions, doctors resort to injections. Vegetarians, please note.

B-12 occurs in microscopic amounts in foods (remember how only a few crystals were isolated from tons of liver). Its weight is measured, not in milligrams, as are other vitamins, but in micrograms (a microgram is 1/1,000 of a milligram). It cannot be made synthetically, but must be grown, like penicillin, in friendly bacteria or molds. Animal protein is almost the only source where it occurs naturally in foods in sufficient amounts. Liver is the best source; kidney, muscle meats, fish and dairy products (milk, milk powder, eggs and cheese) are also good sources. It is found only in traces in some other foods, particularly in vegetables, which are a negligible source. Peanuts, seaweed, Concord grapes and soybeans contain some B-12, although raw soybean flour is deficient in B-12 and creates a need for more vitamin B-12. Wheat germ contains some B-12, and brewer's yeast only if the yeast is bred specifically to include it. B-12 has been found in molded cheese, such as Roquefort, and has been found to increase 15 percent during a three-month cheese-ripening process. Desiccated liver and fresh liver are perhaps the most dependable sources of B-12. Vegetables are not a dependable source.

Adelle Davis wrote: "Vegetarians are particularly subject to pernicious anemia unless they eat generous amounts of milk and eggs. People who have followed a vegetarian diet without milk or eggs for five years or longer often develop sore mouths and tongues, menstrual disturbances and a variety of nervous symptoms including a 'needles and pins' feeling in hands and feet, neuritis, pain and stiffness in the spine and difficulty in walking. All of these symptoms, which are danger signals, dramatically clear up provided B-12 is obtained."[3]

This warning explains why Carlton Fredericks, Ph.D., and other nutritionists urge people to eat some animal protein (or dairy product) with each meal.

Even this precaution may not insure protection, once serious symptoms have set in. Vitamin B-12-deficient people lack one or more substances in the stomach for its absorption. There has long existed a belief that an "intrinsic factor" derived from an animal stomach is a must for those afflicted with pernicious anemia. Without it, the vitamin has appeared to be ineffectual. Although the belief still persists, the intrinsic factor is now available by *prescription only*.

Dr. Fredericks reports that the reason vitamin B-12 is utilized with such great difficulty is that the molecule is so large it does not pass easily through the tiny openings in the intestines and thus may not be absorbed. He states that the body creates its own intrinsic factor, too, providing calcium or magnesium are present in the intestines. He says: "When an individual has difficulty in utilizing vitamin B-12 by mouth, administration by a physician of intrinsic factor or dried stomach tissue (dried under vacuum) and calcium and magnesium would be advisable."[4]

Another discovery is that the use of gastric juice may aid in the absorption of B-12 given orally.[5] And the size of the dose of B-12 may have a bearing on the problem. A Russian study found that whether B-12 was given by mouth in supplement form or by injection, it was more efficiently utilized when provided in small successive doses, rather than in one massive dose.[6] Still another finding is that the thyroid helps B-12 to be better absorbed.[7]

Miss Davis wrote: "Provided iron and vitamin C are obtained with hydrochloric acid, they stimulate the production of the intrinsic factor sufficiently so that persons with mild pernicious anemia can take smaller doses."[8]

The size of the supplemented dose needed for human requirement is unknown. Large amounts are usually given by injection. As little as one microgram may be sufficient providing it is absorbed, according to Bicknell and Prescott.[9] These researchers also state that B-12 "is virtually nontoxic even in a dose ten million times the therapeutic dose." Studies show that what is not used is excreted. Apparently the problem of assimilation is more important than the size of the dose.

Miss Davis added: "If individuals with pernicious anemia who take hydrochloric acid with each meal to assure the absorption of nutrients were to adhere to a completely adequate diet . . . the reverse (of symptoms) could probably be shown."[10]

Bicknell and Prescott add: "At least 100 ml. of normal gastric juice is needed to ensure an adequate response from 1 to 2 micrograms of vitamin B-12 given orally."[11] This would add up to much larger amounts of gastric juice if more B-12 is taken orally.

Miss Davis warned: "To prevent permanent damage, persons adhering to a strict vegetarian diet should probably take 50 micrograms of B-12 each week while their stomach secretions are still normal."[12]

If the symptoms of B-12 deficiencies have become serious, do not try to treat yourself! Rush to the nearest physician for B-12 injections. He will know the amounts to give you. Leave it in his hands.

For prevention, be sure you are taking the entire B complex, which includes B-12, as well as the natural foods, such as those mentioned above. On the label of vitamin supplements, the vitamin may not be listed as B-12, but as cobalamin, or cynocobalamin, both synonyms. But if you are a vegetarian, do not wait for symptoms of B-12 deficiency to become apparent. As Miss Davis wrote: "Because a vegetarian diet is rich in folic acid, however, the blood remains normal and irreparable nerve damage can occur before the vitamin B-12 deficiency is discovered."[13]

Because folic acid can cover up or hide the adverse effects of a B-12 deficiency, folic acid in higher potencies than 0.1 mg. (100 micrograms) per tablet is available only by medical prescription. Let's look at folic acid, another B vitamin, to see what part it plays as a co-worker with B-12, as well as playing its own vital role in several important ailments.

FOLIC ACID

Folic acid was given its name by Dr. Roger J. Williams. It is apparently needed for every cell in the body.[14] It is especially needed for red cell formation. A deficiency of folic acid does cause a certain type of "large cell" anemia, which cannot be corrected by iron. It can occur in pregnant women, in people who do not have enough hydrochloric acid, in children who have suffered from infections, and in anyone who relies upon a refined diet or drinks too much alcohol.[15] Bicknell and Prescott do not believe that folic acid should be used for continuous treatment of pernicious anemia; there may be a relapse and the dose would have to be raised.[16]

However, Dr. Williams, who has done pioneer work on folic acid, assures us that if one receives enough B-12, either by injection or mouth, plus the necessary digestive substances, extra folic acid is harmless.[17] The warning on the label of folic acid available without prescription—"Do not exceed the dose" (0.1 mg. per tablet)—is required by law. For the folic acid available by prescription only, the dosage is usually at least 5 mg. per tablet.

But folic acid is not limited to the treatment of anemia. Its need is indicated in diarrhea, sprue, dropsy, stomach ulcers and menstrual problems. It has repaired leg ulcers[18] and reversed glossitis (tongue inflammation). It, too, has been found to be a factor in mental disease. Dr. Williams also reports a study of seventeen elderly patients afflicted with atherosclerosis (hardening of the arteries) treated with 5 to 7.5 mg. of folic acid daily. Circulation improved, as well as vision.[19] Adelle Davis added that folic acid, if used with some of the other B vitamins (to be discussed in a later chapter), reversed or prevented gray hair in some instances. "The Pill" is an antagonist to folic acid.

Dr. Williams tells of his experience in using folic acid on himself for atherosclerosis, symptoms of which included shortness of breath when walking. He had also suffered from an affliction of one eye. He was already taking a nutritional supplement plus vitamins C and E in substantial amounts. He decided to add magnesium, vitamin B-6 and folic acid to his regime. The result was most encouraging. He developed more vigor, could walk with greater ease and less shortness of breath, improved his golf score and increased his work load to a prodigious level without a feeling of strain. He suddenly realized that he could tolerate cooler temperatures with ease, undoubtedly due to improved circulation. These improvements required several months to become noticeable. Best of all, his affected eye, tested regularly over a period of two months, responded. He says: "I could read about two lines farther down the ophthalmologist's testing chart than before."[20]

Apparently a deficiency of folic acid is not unusual, but widespread. And there seems to be little concern over toxicity resulting from taking it as a supplement. An English study reported that twenty young healthy adults were given 15 mg. of folic acid and matched with a control group given placebos, for one month. No ill effect was found of the use of folic acid.[21] As a matter of fact, physicians have given 150 mg. of folic acid to children and 450 mg. to adults, both daily, and report no toxicity at all.[22] Many nutritionists feel that it is unfortunate that this vitamin has been put on the prescription list in potencies no higher than 0.1 mg. per tablet. Adelle Davis stated firmly: "Were 5 mg. of folic acid added with vitamin B-12 to supplements, vegetarians, as well as most other persons, could be protected, though some few require 20 mg. of folic acid daily.[23]

For some mysterious reason, folic acid in 5 mg. potency, formerly available at pharmacies without a prescription, has disappeared from the druggist shelves in the United States. Is it banned by the FDA or the AMA or both? No one seems to know.

According to *Health Food Retailing* (December, 1972), the AMA still believes in it. Here is the HFR story:

"The Journal of the American Medical Association for July 31, 1972, reports on the case of a sixty-nine-year-old woman who was brought to a hospital with a history of pallor, fatigue, forgetfulness and lack of energy. On the day before, she fell in her apartment and was unable to get up. Hospital attendants found it difficult to awaken her.

"After thorough tests, it was obvious that she was suffering from megaloblastic anemia, with diseased red blood cells and other symptoms characteristic of the anemia caused by lack of vitamin B-12. But she had received an injection of vitamin B-12 a week before she came to the hospital, and her blood levels of this vitamin were high.

"Then the doctors gave her folic acid, a B vitamin closely related to vitamin B-12. She began to improve at once and was soon discharged from the hospital. Tests six months later showed her in good health. Her mind was clear, she walked normally, and her fatigue and forgetfulness were gone.

"The authors of the JAMA article note that this patient came from a family where there was a history of pernicious anemia. They also report that two other elderly patients were cured of their 'dementia' with folic acid."

Except for the problem of folic acid covering up a deficiency of B-12 in the body, the only other contra-indication I found in the literature was in connection with cancer and leukemia. Some researchers believe that folic acid hastens the development of leukemia; others feel it does not make the disease worse, but instead improves the well-being of the patient.[24] Although folic acid inhibits some kinds of cancer in rats,[25] in humans, once cancer is present, folic acid is questionable.[26] As late as 1962, the date of the third edition of their textbook, Bicknell and Prescott said: "Folic acid is required by the monkey, fox, chick, dog, rat, guinea pig, turkey, mosquito and certain microorganisms. . . . In man, the human requirement is purely conjectural."[27]

Let us not worry too much over the concern in some quarters about folic acid. As long as you are taking B-12 simultaneously, as well as foods such as brewer's yeast and liver in some form to supply all of the other B vitamins, the supplements of folic acid are considered both safe and helpful. What foods contain folic acid in liberal amounts? Here is a list:[28] Fresh, dark green leafy vegetables and liver are rich sources. Cauliflower, kidney and chicken giblets contain it too, in fair amounts. But cooking and long storage create losses. (Refrigerated food can contain folic acid up to two weeks only.) Prolonged cooking of cabbage was found to destroy all its folic acid (37 to 94 percent was leached into the water, which most people pour down the sink) . . .

To give you an idea of the amount of folic acid in foods (measured in micrograms), there are:

98 micrograms of folic acid in one-half cup of mushrooms

140–160 micrograms of folic acid in six tablespoons of wheat germ

280 micrograms of folic acid in two slices of liver

1,040 micrograms of folic acid in three tablespoons of brewer's yeast

Remember that these last three foods also contain the other B vitamins (B-12 is in yeast only if bred to include it, so read your labels.) It is no accident that these three foods are often referred to as the "wonder foods" despite the disparaging remarks of those who refuse to acknowledge the value of nutrition.

Vitamin B-12 has at last been completely synthesized in the laboratory. The synthetic cyanocobalamin is used to aid blood formation, nerve function and various metabolic processes in which it acts as a coenzyme. Its synthesis is the result of the work of ninety-nine scientists in nineteen countries during eleven years. It is a chelated form of cobalt. When used orally, it must be associated with the gastric intrinsic factor to make it effective.[29]

REFERENCES

1. *Canadian Medical Association Journal.* February 28, 1970.

2. Roger J. Williams, Ph.D. *Nutrition Against Disease.* Paperback edition. New York: Bantam, 1973.

3. Adelle Davis. *Let's Get Well.* Paperback edition. New York: New American Library, 1972.

4. *The Carlton Fredericks Newsletter of Nutrition.* Vol. 1, No. 12, December 15, 1971.

5. J. I. Rodale and Staff. *The Complete Book of Nutrition*. Emmaus, Pa.: Rodale Books, 1966.

6. *Nutritional Abstracts and Reviews*. April, 1957, p. 389.

7. *Nutritional Abstracts and Reviews*. October, 1961, Abstract No. 5510.

8. Adelle Davis, *op. cit.*

9. Bicknell and Prescott. *The Vitamins in Medicine*. Third Edition. Milwaukee, Wis. 53201: Lee Foundation for Nutritional Research, 1962.

10. Adelle Davis, *op. cit.*

11. Bicknell and Prescott, *op. cit.*

12. Adelle Davis, *op. cit.*

13. Adelle Davis, *op. cit.*

14. Roger J. Williams, *op. cit.*

15. Adelle Davis, *op. cit.*

16. Bicknell and Prescott, *op. cit.*

17. Roger J. Williams, *op. cit.*

18. *Nutritional Abstracts and Reviews*. January, 1969, Abstract No. 1197.

19. Roger J. Williams, *op. cit.*

20. Roger J. Williams, *op. cit.*

21. *Lancet*. Vol. 1, pp. 59–61, 1971.

22. Adelle Davis, *op. cit.*

23. Adelle Davis, *op. cit.*

24. Adelle Davis, *op. cit.*

25. J. I. Rodale, *op. cit.*

26. Roger J. Williams, *op. cit.*

27. Bicknell and Prescott, *op. cit.*

28. J. I. Rodale, *op. cit.*

29. *Science*. Vol. 179, p. 166, 1973.

11
Choline and Inositol

In these days of great concern about cholesterol and fats, have you ever wished for a detergent that could dissolve the cholesterol and fatty deposits in certain parts of your body? Many people (even doctors) are laboring under the misapprehension that if you avoid eating cholesterol, you can avoid cholesterol deposits. Not so. This information is sadly out of date. The body manufactures cholesterol whether you eat it or not, and some of the high cholesterol foods, including eggs, are the finest foods known. The body actually needs them. There are a variety of other reasons why cholesterol may pile up in the body, and these deposits can be handled successfully—not by avoiding cholesterol foods, but by using one or more nutrients that can emulsify or dissolve such deposits. Albert E. Holand, Jr., describes one of these substances as a "detergent." It is not a household detergent of course, but a vitamin-like substance that does the job. It is considered a member of the B vitamin family and is called choline.[1]

Actually, according to Holand, from a strictly technical point of view it is not a vitamin at all, for two reasons: (a) choline can be manufactured in the body if certain other substances are present, and (b) much more choline is needed than the average vitamin.

The name "choline" is derived from the Greek word *cholera*, which means "bile," from which choline has been isolated. Gallstones can be produced by very high concentrations of cholesterol, also found in bile. But if there is sufficient choline, it can emulsify or dissolve the waxlike cholesterol and is capable of preventing gallstones. Holand finds that choline is excellent for biliousness, certain types of digestive upsets, particularly those related to the assimilation of fats that result in a pale, pasty complexion. He says: "I have seen many bilious-appearing persons take on a fresh, rosy appearance after the use of choline, which I attribute to an improvement in the capillary circulation as well as in liver and gall bladder function."

Adelle Davis agreed. She found that weak capillary walls are strengthened by choline. For this reason, it appears to be successful in reducing high blood pressure. She quoted the results of a study of a group of patients whose blood pressure has been dangerously high. The symptoms of heart palpitation, dizziness, headaches, ear noises—even constipation—were either relieved or disappeared entirely within five to ten days after choline was given. Insomnia and visual disturbances were relieved, too, and the blood flow to the eyes improved steadily over a two-year period. But, when choline therapy was stopped, the capillary walls again became weak and the blood pressure often increased. As long as the choline treatment was continued, the blood pressure dropped to normal in more than a third of the patients.[2]

Because choline is a fat and cholesterol emulsifier, or dissolver, or detergent (its technical name is "lipotropic agent"), it is used for atherosclerosis, or fatty congestion of the arteries. It is also used for fatty livers, liver damage, cirrhosis of the liver and hepatitis. It is used in kidney damage, hemorrhaging of the kidneys and nephritis, as well as for such eye conditions as ocular hemorrhages and glaucoma. It appears to be, among other factors, a cancer preventive. In one study, fourteen out of eighteen rats not fed choline developed cancer, whereas in a group of rats fed choline, none developed the disease.[3] Choline has also proved to be a shield against some toxic drugs.[4]

Wouldn't you think this was about enough to expect from one lone nutrient? But these are by no means all of the benefits that result from the use of choline. It also plays a part in preventing or reversing muscle weakness, especially in myasthenia gravis. In one of my books, I told of a man who overcame this disease by using lecithin. Is there any connection between choline and lecithin? Indeed there is. Choline was first found in brain lecithin. This is why the choline-rich lecithin has been found to dissolve or lower cholesterol levels.[5]

What other foods contain choline? Choline is found in liver and yeast and in extremely high amounts in egg yolks. (How foolish to forbid them in the diet.) As many as twelve eggs per day have been eaten without causing a cholesterol rise, providing the eggs were not cooked in hydrogenated fat. And this scare over butterfat is just as unnecessary. Scandinavian countries eat far more butterfat than Americans and have lower cholesterol levels and less heart disease. As Miss Davis said: "In the days when atherosclerosis was unheard of in America, butter was slathered in or on every food not cooked in cream. But·

terfat appears to be a problem only when nutrients needed to utilize it are undersupplied."[6] These necessary nutrients include choline and lecithin. One study revealed that taking one ounce of lecithin a day dissolved cholesterol deposits.[7] Choline-rich lecithin, a derivative of soy beans, can be taken in granule or liquid form. It can also be manufactured in the body, but not unless vitamin B-6 and magnesium are present. Methionine (an amino acid or protein factor), plus a high protein diet, as well as folic acid and vitamin B-12, are also necessary for its manu facture.

How much choline should one take separately in supplement form? Or can you get enough in food sources? Carlton Fredericks, Ph.D., believes it is better to play safe and get enough through supplements. He takes 1,000 mg. (1 gram) of choline daily. According to Bicknell and Prescott, a toxic dose is not reached until it exceeds 6,000 mg. (6 gm.).[8] These researchers do suggest that the choline should be taken in divided doses (with each meal), rather than all at once. And there is evidence that choline can induce a deficiency of vitamin B-6.[9] So we come to the old warning again about taking too much of one B vitamin without the others. To avoid an imbalance, take a food *rich in all the B vitamins* together with the supplement of any separate B vitamin needed. Liver and yeast in clude all the B vitamins, excepting B-12, unless the yeast is specifically bred to include it. Reading labels will help you to find such a yeast, as suggested in the preceding chapter.

Dr. Fredericks says: "Choline is more effective when accompanied by inositol, another B vitamin, and other vitamins that affect fat utilization."

INOSITOL

Just because you may have heard little about inositol, don't sell it short. Actually, little is known about it, but it is another fat dissolver and acts as a partner to choline. Inositol does some things choline doesn't, however. For example, it can be a factor in reducing. And it has won praise in many cases by its effect on falling hair. We have learned in previous chapters that B-6 and folic acid help prevent thinning hair, but Adelle Davis specifically recommended inositol in substantial amounts to men becoming bald.[10] Inositol is also found to be helpful in brain cell nutrition, and has been recommended in this connection by Dr. Abram Hoffer, famed, as mentioned earlier, for his megavitamin therapy for schizophrenia and other forms of mental illness.[11]

Inositol is needed for the growth and cell survival in bone marrow, eye membranes and intestines. It is found in large amounts in various areas of the body: brain, stomach, kidney, spleen, liver, heart, thyroid and human hair, showing that it is needed nutritionally to keep the supply up to normal levels. As Dr. Williams says: ". . . An animal or human being may be benefited by an added amount in the diet."[11]

Where can you find inositol? It is present in most plant and animal sources, particularly in fruits and cereals. But, unfortunately, it is removed from most foods by processing. Because of this, Dr. Fredericks states that he uses daily supplements of inositol of several hundred mg. Liver and brewer's yeast are rich sources of inositol. One analysis of yeast shows that, in addition to the other B vitamins, as well as many minerals and amino acids for protein, one tablespoon of yeast provides 40 mg. each of choline and inositol.

Now you can begin to see why the B vitamins are so fantastic. Each one seems to outdo the other. In the next chapter we'll discuss three more: pantothenic acid, PABA and biotin.

REFERENCES

1. Albert E. Holand, Jr. *Importance of Creative Nutrition,* 1971. Available only from Ectolyte Products, 13169-A Brookhurst Street, Garden Grove, Calif. 92643.

2. Adelle Davis. *Let's Get Well.* Paperback edition. New York: New American Library, 1972.

3. Roger J. Williams. *Nutrition Against Disease.* Paperback edition. New York: Bantam, 1973.

4. Adelle Davis, *op. cit.*

5. Roger J. Williams, *op. cit.*

6. Adelle Davis, *op. cit.*

7. Roger J. Williams, *op. cit.*

8. Bicknell and Prescott. *The Vitamins in Medicine.* Milwaukee, Wis.: Lee Foundation for Nutritional Research, 1962.

9. *Nutrition Abstracts and Reviews.* April, 1968, Abstract No. 2505.

10. Adelle Davis, *op. cit.*

11. Roger J. Williams, *op. cit.*

12. Roger J. Williams, *op. cit.*

See also:

Carl C. Pfeiffer and Jane Banks. "C—Inositol—B6: The Sleepy Threesome." *Health Quarterly,* Nov./Dec. 1980.

12
Pantothenic Acid, PABA and Biotin

A friend called recently and told me with elation: "My beauty operator told me today that my hair has thickened up unbelievably during the last six months and is also more lustrous and manageable. Knowing I am interested in nutrition, she asked what I was taking. I told her the only new nutrient I had added to my diet was pantothenic acid. I began it just six months ago."

This report, though admittedly only one case, surprised me. Pantothenic acid has been credited with other types of hair improvement, as you will see, but it is primarily noted as an antistress vitamin. My friend, whose hair was apparently improved by it, is not a stress-prone person. It is true that when pantothenic acid was given to rats deficient in this B vitamin, if the animals were bald, or had gray hair, the symptoms were reversed and hair even turned black. Wrinkled skin and skin ulcers, considered symptoms of aging, were also reversed by pantothenic acid.

Dr. Agnes Fay Morgan, formerly of the University of

California at Berkeley, is famed for her experiment with animals whose prematurely gray hair was found to be caused by damaged adrenal glands. When the glands were repaired by the administration of pantothenic acid, the hair returned to its original color. Not all humans are as lucky, however.

Pantothenic acid was discovered by Dr. Roger J. Williams. The name is derived from the Greek word *panthos*, meaning "universal" or "from everywhere." Pantothenic acid occurs in all living cells. Its greatest contribution, known to date, is its effect on the adrenal cortex, which, due to a pantothenic acid deficiency, can result in allergies, low resistance to stress, some forms of arthritis, gout and a high level of uric acid, sore throat, quick temper, breathlessness, muscular weakness, overwhelming fatigue and a disturbed pulse rate.

Many physicians give patients with these symptoms of adrenal exhaustion, cortisone or its derivatives (which should be manufactured by the body itself). Unfortunately, these drugs can create drastic side effects, including growth of facial hair and a swelling of the face known as "moon face." Since pantothenic acid is a vitamin, needed by the adrenal glands, according to other physicians, it is far safer to use the vitamin rather than the questionable drugs. Dr. T. Ogawa, writing in a medical journal, says it is possible to get the same good effects from pantothenic acid, without the toxic effects produced by ACTH or cortisone.[1]

Adelle Davis wrote: "Any form of stress exhausts the supply of pantothenic acid. Yet," she continued, "when plenty of pantothenic acid is taken, if the deprivation has not been too prolonged, the body begins producing its own natural hormones in as short a time as twenty-four hours. Of course, if the deficiency has been present for a long time, recovery is slower."[2]

For example, when volunteers were deprived of pantothenic acid for just a short time, all of them displayed such reactions as muscular weakness, cramps, poor coordination and hand tremors. Prisoners in Iowa State Prison, who were given a good diet except for pantothenic acid, developed low blood pressure, dizziness, extreme fatigue, respiratory infections, muscular weakness, stomach distress and constipation. Yet, when pantothenic acid was given them daily, many recovered in three weeks.[3]

Pantothenic acid also has some other surprises. A mild deficiency can result in a reduction of hydrochloric acid, needed for digestion of protein and minerals; if the deficiency becomes severe, the hydrochloric acid manufacture may go to the opposite extreme of too much acid, inducing ulcers.[4] Pantothenic acid has also been used to prevent radiation damage in mice and protect people against allergy.[5]

Arthritis can result from adrenal exhaustion. Dr. Williams states that pantothenic acid may be important in preventing arthritis. He found the average level of pantothenic acid for arthritic patients to be about 65 percent of that of well people. Severely crippled people were found to have only 40 percent of the normal pantothenic acid level; two of these were bedridden.[6] Adelle Davis cited the cases of several arthritics who were given small doses of pantothenic acid as their only dietary addition. Some experienced a decrease of pain and stiffness within weeks. However, Dr. Williams quotes one study in which pantothenic acid brought relief in arthritis after seven days, but further improvement did not continue. The conclusion was that pantothenic acid may not be the complete answer; other essential factors are also involved. As Dr. Williams says: "The whole nutritional chain of life is needed by cells with a deficient environment."[7] In other words, the body needs not just one, but all nutrients for health.

Dr. Williams does give pantothenic acid credit for success with mental disease. And a test with human volunteers showed that pantothenic acid prevented a rise in blood sugar. This would fit into hypoglycemia therapy. One physician, Alan H. Nittler, M.D., who specializes in this disease, believes that the adrenal glands are often involved. Dr. Williams believes that vitamins should be used as a team, not singly. This certainly applies to the B complex.

Dr. Williams, the "father" of pantothenic acid, states that one of the uses of pantothenic acid is to help develop general good health; but, as mentioned previously, he cautions that it should be combined with a source of *all* B vitamins.

He lists other benefits of pantothenic acid:

A protection against damage to the adrenal cortex, which can result from pantothenic acid deficiency

Maintenance of a healthy digestive tract

Prevention of nerve degeneration due to pantothenic deficiency (This includes peripheral neuritis, nerve disorders and epilepsy.)

Water balance in the body

Brain and memory improvement

He adds that because, like other B vitamins, pantothenic acid is essential to every cell in the body, the following pathological conditions have resulted in animals from its deficiency:

Skin and hair disturbances

Ulcers
Anemia
Fatty liver
Hemorrhage and necrosis of kidneys
Sciatic nerve and spinal cord degeneration
Mottled thymus
Heart damage
Atrophy of the adrenals
Spinal curvature

Dr. Williams states that the pantothenic acid requirement is far greater than that for vitamins B-1 and B-2. He adds that 100 mg. of pantothenic acid daily has never been found toxic.

Dr. Williams makes a very important point in connection with any vitamin: "It should not be taken for granted that vitamin deficiencies may arise only because of an incomplete diet . . . [but] because of some metabolic disturbance, or an infection, which causes relatively rapid destruction or excretion of a vitamin or prevents its normal absorption."[8]

Pantothenic acid is usually sold as calcium pantothenate. What is the amount that should be used? The daily requirement has not been established. Tests on animals show that human needs vary. One source suggests 5 to 10 mg. daily. Others 50 to 100 mg. daily. In one study, 1,000 mg. daily. No toxic effects have been experienced even when 500 times the amounts recommended by the National Research Council have been given.

What foods contain pantothenic acid? Codfish ovaries, royal jelly (an extremely rich source), pecans, peanuts, egg yolk, wheat germ, brown rice, eggs, mushrooms and the most dependable sources of pantothenic acid: liver and yeast. Folic acid is said to help the assimilation of pantothenic acid. Pantothenic acid has been used in a formula including two other B vitamins for reversing hair color in some instances. One of these vitamins is PABA, which we will discuss next.

PABA

PABA is an abbreviation for a jawbreaker: Para-Amino-Benzoic acid, another B vitamin. It is a recently discovered vitamin, if it is a vitamin at all. In 1942, the government decided it was a B vitamin and criticized any vitamin B complex mixture that did not contain it. A short year later, they reversed themselves and decided that PABA was neither a vitamin, nor a drug, but a chemical.

There is still much controversy about PABA. Even though most people now consider it a B vitamin, there is much argument about its effects. Researchers cannot agree whether or not it can recolor prematurely gray hair, and whether or not it is also useful in vitiligo, that peculiar disturbance in which small patches of skin turn white, or at least lose their color. There is documented evidence that PABA can be a help for vitiligo,[9] as well as for hair recoloring, although Bicknell and Prescott state that earlier studies have never been repeated or proved.[10] One physician, H. W. Francis, M.D., discovered that when an absence of hydrochloric acid was corrected, vitiligo disappeared.[11]

What everyone does agree upon is that PABA is an antagonist to the sulfa drugs, once so popular, but which have since been reported as being a dangerous type of antibiotic. When sulfa is given, PABA apparently cannot function in the body; and folic acid synthesis in the intestines, which helps the assimilation of pantothenic acid, is disturbed, thus putting three vitamins (pantothenic acid, folic acid and PABA) out of commission simultaneously.[12] When this happens, digestive disturbances, nervousness and depression follow. Because of this inactivating effect of PABA against the sulfa drugs (which are rarely used anymore), potencies of PABA higher than 30 mg. per tablet are available only by prescription. The PABA antagonism to sulfa drugs is given as the reason for this action. However, I find another reason why PABA may be a prescription item. According to Bicknell and Prescott, although PABA can have good results, it can be toxic for heart, kidney, and liver. Toxic hepatitis has been reported following its administration. According to these doctors: "A warning is necessary against the continuous ingestion of PABA."[13] This would not apply to PABA-rich foods.

There is no argument over the fact that PABA, when added to a salve and applied to the skin, may protect against sunburn, and even prevent skin cancer.[14]

PABA is also considered helpful, when used in creams, for a variety of skin disturbances, including eczemas and lupus erythematosus. Bicknell and Prescott have included before-and-after pictures of such improvement in their textbook.[15]

PABA is water-soluble. It is not stored in the tissues, but is synthesized by friendly bacteria in the intestines. This means that if conditions are favorable, we can manufacture our own. PABA also occurs plentifully in liver, brewer's yeast, milk, yogurt, eggs, whole rice and cereals, wholewheat, wheat germ and molasses, and in lesser amounts in beef and pork.[16] It is removed by processing from most foods. There is agreement that, especially in the case of PABA, the other B factors in natural foods should also be added.

PABA is one of the nutrients reported to have been successful in recoloring gray hair (the other nutrients are copper, folic acid, and pantothenic acid). Many years ago, Dr. Benjamin Sieve of Boston gave PABA to 300 patients of both sexes, ages sixteen to seventy-four, with gray or graying hair, which had existed for from two to twenty-four years. The patients noted a change in their hair color usually within the first five weeks of treatment. First a yellowish cast and then a somewhat dirty color appeared in the hair of those who had been blond. A dark, dusty gray appeared in the hair of the persons formerly brunettes. Then there was a gradual return to the normal color. Increase in hair lustre and health were also noted. The time required for the complete change seemed to depend upon the physical condition of the person. Three-fourths of Dr. Sieve's patients achieved success, he reported.

Dr. Sieve gave PABA straight. Another physician, using another B vitamin on prisoners, had better success. Dr. Carlton Fredericks decided to combine all the factors tested into a hair recoloring formula. This included 100 mg. of PABA, 30 mg. of pantothenic acid and 2,000 mg. of choline. This formula changed flamingo feathers from faded pink to red, as well as changing the hair color of some people. Dr. Fredericks says that it may have taken a long time to acquire gray hair and he suggests not expecting results in less than six months.[17]

Adelle Davis stated that PABA used alone has, in some cases, restored the natural hair color, but she added: "I have seen many instances of gray hair that returned temporarily to its original color, but it quickly becomes gray again unless one continues to eat yogurt, liver, yeast, and wheat germ."[18] She left out blackstrap molasses. I have reported in two of my books of a man who reversed his hair color with blackstrap, and this has been repeated by other people who followed the procedure faithfully and consistently.[19,20] There is no mystery about this: blackstrap molasses contains a number of the B vitamins, including pantothenic acid, as well as copper, which is needed for the assimilation of iron. Taking copper or any other vitamin B nutrient separately is a questionable practice. I have known of people suffering from copper poisoning by getting too much. But taking minerals or the B vitamin in a natural food is an entirely different matter, and appears to supply protection against nutritional imbalance.

BIOTIN

Biotin is another perplexing vitamin. It appears in small quantities in all animal and plant tissue. It appears in our bodies in microscopic amounts. Like B-12, it is needlelike in structure. It is measured not in milligrams but in micrograms or far smaller potencies. Biotin must be present in the body, even in infinitesimal amounts, or trouble results. If it is lacking, skin problems such as pallor, eczema, dermatitis and hair loss may occur (though hair loss may occur from a lack of almost any nutrient).

Biotin deficiency is uncommon, but when its deficiency is induced, depression, lassitude, hallucinations and panic may occur. When it is supplied, these symptoms cease.[21] One means of producing a biotin deficiency in animals is by giving them large amounts of raw egg white, which contains avidin, an antagonist to biotin. But there is no need to panic. According to J. D. Walters, M.D., raw infertile egg white is hard for many people to assimilate, whereas he believes that raw fertile egg is easily tolerated by most people.[22] Also, one study revealed that when a group of human patients were fed the raw whites of thirty-six to forty-two eggs daily for a year, their general condition actually improved.[23] J. I. Rodale comments that in laboratory experiments, the egg white was given without the yolks.[24] Few people eat just the white of egg, and the whole egg may be needed for balance of the nutrients included. This has certainly proved to be true in other foods: for example, beri-beri resulting from rice that has had its coating removed. No problem has been found in eating the whole food, instead of the separated factors.

Biotin is another nutrient, which, if our intestinal flora is in optimum condition, we can manufacture ourselves. If, however, you have resorted to antibiotics or drugs that kill the friendly flora, you may need soured milks or acidophilus added to your diet until the intestines are again normal. Biotin deficiency is not to be feared if you include in your diet such foods as brewer's yeast, liver, kidney, unpolished rice, soy flour, soy beans, egg yolks and green vegetables.

We are coming to the end of the line for the B vitamins. We will finish this family, or complex, in the next chapter with the discussion of the controversial B-15 and B-17.

REFERENCES

1. *American Journal of Physiology*. Vol. 198, p. 619, 1960.

2. Adelle Davis. *Let's Get Well*. Paperback edition. New York: New American Library, 1972.

3. *Ibid*.

4. *Ibid*.

5. *Acta. Ped. Hunga.*, 1963.

6. Roger J. Williams. *Nutrition Against Disease.* Paperback edition. New York: Bantam, 1973.

7. *Ibid.*

8. *Ibid.*

9. Adelle Davis, *op. cit.*

10. Bicknell and Prescott. *The Vitamin in Medicine.* Milwaukee, Wis.: Lee Foundation for Nutritional Research, 1962.

11. J. I. Rodale and staff. *The Complete Book of Vitamins.* Emmaus, Pa.: Rodale Books, 1966.

12. *Ibid.*

13. Bicknell and Prescott, *op. cit.*

14. Adelle Davis, *op. cit.*

15. Bicknell and Prescott, *op. cit.*

16. J. I. Rodale and staff, *op. cit.*

17. Linda Clark. *Stay Young Longer.* Paperback edition. New York: Pyramid Communications, 1968.

18. Adelle Davis, *op. cit.*

19. Linda Clark, *op. cit.*

20. Linda Clark. *Secrets of Health and Beauty.* Paperback edition. New York: Berkley-Jove, 1979

21. Roger J. Williams, *op. cit.*

22. Linda Clark. *Get Well Naturally.* Paperback edition. New York: Arco Publishing, 1972.

23. Bicknell and Prescott, *op. cit.*

24. J. I. Rodale and staff, *op. cit.*

See also:

Richard Wentzler. *The Vitamin Book.* New York: St. Martin's Press, 1978.

13
The Controversial
B-15 and B-17

B-15, or pangamic acid, is little known and little used in this country, if it is available at all. This is a great pity because the Russians use it widely, considering it a life-saving vitamin. One U.S. visitor, writing from Russia, said: "We were interested to see vitamins A, B-1, B-2, B-6, B-15, C and calcium tablets in all of the pharmacies. We have found no equivalent of the health store anywhere. . . . A bottle of 100 tablets of B-15, 50 mg. each, costs the equivalent of $1.52. Later, when we were in Ulan Bator, Mongolia, we came across a black market peddler hawking ever so cautiously a single bottle of vitamin B-15. The asking price was $7.50."

Why are the Russians so excited about B-15? Because of its success for many conditions, as reported by researchers: "Among all circulatory problems, heart conditions, elevated blood cholesterol, various skin conditions, emphysema and premature aging."[1]

A study conducted in Russia on forty-two cases supplies further information and explains why the Russians regard B-15 with great respect. The study[2] states: "B-15, in the form of calcium pangamate, was prescribed for oral use, 30 mg. three times daily, or a total of 90 mg. daily. The treatment lasted twenty days.

"At the end of the twenty days, all our patients showed improvement in their clinical condition. The pains in the heart area, shortness of breath, weakness and cyanosis of the mucous membrane of the lips subsided or disappeared. In cases of marked tachycardia (rapid pulse) a decrease of the number of contractions was noticed, while in the cases of moderate or insignificant tachycardia the conditions changed to absolute normal state . . .

"In all six cases of circulatory disturbance the liver had reached its normal size at the end of the treatment with B-15 . . .

"The general cholesterol content was examined in all forty-two cases. It was measured before treatment, after ten days of treatment, and at the end of the twenty days of treatment. Before treatment the general level of cholesterol averaged 211 . . . after twenty days of treatment, 175 . . . In most cases the drop of the cholesterol was noticed as early as ten days after beginning the treatment and continued over the following period. Ten days after the end of the treatment with vitamin B-15, the general level of cholesterol was 163. We have noticed that the higher the cholesterol was at the beginning of the treatment, the more it dropped due to the action of B-15."

Research on B-15 reveals that the vitamin supplies oxygen to the cells and the heart. It also acts as a detoxicant. When alcoholics were treated with B-15, they lost their craving for alcohol. One-half of the patients addicted to narcotics also responded. B-15 has been found helpful, too, in chronic hepatitis and early liver cirrhosis.

Findings by N. Yakovlev, a worker at the Institute of Physical Culture in Russia, shows evidence that B-15 improves physical energy.[3]

Vitamin B-15 has been found helpful in early healing of muscles of injured legs.[4] Groups of athletes have been given various amounts of various substances to stimulate energy in muscular activity. The results of these studies indicated that 300 mg. of B-15 on successive days was the most effective.[5]

The Russians have combined vitamins A, E and B-15 into an allegedly miracle-performing product they call Aevit. It was used in one clinic with patients who were, on their arrival, candidates for leg amputation. These patients ranged from fifty to ninety-five years in age and had developed gangrene. Within two months they started walking again. Of 203 patients with obliterating atherosclerosis (a form of hardening of the arteries) of the lower limbs, 180 were discharged, practically healthy. One man previously condemned by surgeons to amputation of both legs was photographed jumping over a fence only a few months after beginning the treatment. He was shown with a Professor Shpirt, a researcher in this clinic, who reported to the conference at the Institute of Biochemistry: "I believe the time will come when there will be calcium pangamate (B-15) next to the saltcellar on the table of every family with people past forty."[6]

B-15, or pangamic acid, was originally isolated by the late Ernst T. Krebs, M.D., and his son, E. T. Krebs, Jr., of San Francisco. It is a water-soluble substance found in apricot kernels and other seeds, as well as in rice bran and polish, whole grain cereals, brewer's yeast, steer blood and horse liver. It is nontoxic.

You may or may not be able to buy vitamin B-15, since it has been on and off the market in this country.

Not only Russia is far ahead of us in its use of B-15; there are four or five ethical brands of B-15 in Germany available to the public. The explanation given by the FDA in this country is that it is not considered dangerous, merely ineffective. Russian research refutes this attitude. They consider B-15 a *must* for health.

Vitamin B-15 is now being given to Olympic athletes and its use is spreading to many European countries. Recent research of its values, the best type to take and the suggested dosage, appears in a helpful book by Brenda Forman: *B-15, The Miracle Vitamin*, published in 1979, by Fred Jordan Books, Grosset and Dunlap).

VITAMIN B-17

B-17, also known as the nitrilosides, is still more controversial. The medical dosage forms of this vitamin are known as Laetrile. Laetrile has not been accepted as a cancer treatment in the United States. This is not surprising, since no natural unorthodox dosage for cancer has been allowed or even adequately tested in this country. In California, for example, no cancer treatment is considered legal except surgery, radiation and chemotherapy. This explains why Americans are looking for help and hope in other countries. Consequently, 2,500 cancer sufferers who have not been helped by treatments in the U.S. have flocked to Mexico where Laetrile is manufactured and its use is allowed. It is also being manufactured in Monaco. Its originators honestly admit that used alone it does not cure; it mainly controls cancer. When it is combined with other nutrients, however, some "miracles" have resulted.

Again, as in the case of vitamin B-15, vitamin B-17 has been condemned, not because it is dangerous, but because the government insists there is no evidence or proof that it is helpful. Dr. Dean Burk, former head of the cytochemistry section of the National Cancer Institute, has tested Laetrile on mice and states: "The stuff is absolutely harmless, so why not give it a try?"[7]

Ernst T. Krebs, Jr., Ph.D., a biochemist, assures the public that B-17 is totally nontoxic. White rats fed seventy times the normal human dose of B-17 used in the palliation of human cancer were completely normal and healthy after ninety days. None died. The only side effects noticed were greater weight and appetite because they were receiving a nourishing vitamin, not a drug.

B-17 is found in the kernels of practically all fruits: apples, cherries, peaches, plums, nectarines, etc., in the prodigious concentration of 2 to 3 percent. In a personal communication to me, Ernst Krebs, Jr., stated that it has not thus far been found in citrus fruits in this country, although Professor Oke, Department of Chemistry, of the University of Life, Ibadan, Nigeria, reports the traces of B-17 in citrus fruit seeds.

B-17 is also found in sixty-two plant foods and seventy plants used for animal fodder. Sprouted seeds contain ten to thirty times as much B-17 as mature plants. B-17 is one vitamin that does not naturally occur in brewer's yeast.

If you cannot find B-15 or B-17 in single supplementary form, or as a part of a multiple vitamin supplement, where can you get these important vitamins? *From whole, natural foods.* Our ancestors did not have health stores because they did not need them. Every farm and garden served as a household health-food supply. By eating this whole, natural food, they prevented much of the appalling illness so common today. They did not even do it with drugs. There were few drugs then; and those few were derived from natural plant or herb sources, not synthesized in the laboratories.

E. T. Krebs, Jr., says: "The diet of primitive man and most fruit-eating animals was very rich in vitamin B-17. They regularly ate the seeds or kernels of all fruits, since these seeds were rich in protein, unsaturated fats and other nutrients. There are scores of foods naturally or normally very rich in B-17."[8]

Dr. Krebs likes to use the analogy of a person shipwrecked on a tropical isle. If this person consumed the *whole* fruit, together with the seeds which supply 45 percent protein, 40 percent polyunsaturated fats and other nutrients, including minerals—the seeds are high in calcium and magnesium—the castaway could maintain perfect health on this limited whole food fare.

We have encountered this whole food principle before: in the heart disease of the cattle whose fodder had been depleted of vitamin E; in the prisoners and chickens who contracted beri-beri eating rice from which the vitamin B coating had been removed; in the pellagra patients whose cornmeal had been degerminated, thus removing the vital B vitamins. These were rescued with brewer's yeast which contains most of those B vitamins in high amounts.

Food depleted of its natural vitamins and enriched with some synthetic vitamins is not a safe substitute for whole, natural foods. This is witnessed by the study, previously mentioned, in which Dr. Williams reported that rats fed enriched bread died or were severely stunted, due to malnutruion. Rats fed a wholegrain bread flourished.

Much illness, we are learning, may be due to vitamin-mineral deficiencies. Even senility has been proved to be caused by a deficiency of vitamins B and C and more recently vitamin E.[9]

This brings us to the close of the fabulous vitamin B family. There are others being "discovered," such as orotic acid and carnitine, but to date the information of what they accomplish is limited. By eating your whole foods, particularly liver, or desiccated liver, and yeast, you will probably get them anyway.

REFERENCES

1. *Let's Live.* November, 1971.

2. "Physician's New Weapon." A series of research reports and documentation, translated from the Russian language.

3. *Ibid.*

4. *Nutrition Abstracts and Reviews.* July, 1971. Abstract No. 5151.

5. *Nutrition Abstracts and Reviews.* October, 1967. Abstract No. 6251.

6. "Physician's New Weapon," *op. cit.*

7. *Time.* April 12, 1971.

8. E. T. Krebs, Jr. "The Nitrilosides (Vitamin B-17): Their Nature, Occurrence and Metabolic Significance (Antineoplastic B-17)," *Journal of Applied Nutrition.* Vol. 22, Nos. 3 and 4, 1970.

9. Abram Hoffer and Morton Walker. *Nutrients to Age Without Senility.* New Canaan, Conn.: Keats Publishing, Inc., 1980.

14
Vitamin C

There are two general forms of vitamin C: the entire family or complex, known as the bioflavonoids; and a single factor in this family, called ascorbic acid. The bioflavonoids are in natural form; ascorbic acid, synthetic. But ascorbic acid is one synthetic that does its job well. It is also one synthetic vitamin you need not be afraid to take in large and continuous doses, according to physicians and other researchers who have tested it with both success and safety for years. We will discuss the achievements of ascorbic acid first.

If you wish to convert yourself, or anyone else, to the values of nutrition, vitamin C is the vitamin to use as a beginner. It does, as Dr. Linus Pauling has assured us, control the common cold if used properly,[1] and it can accomplish so many other miracles that I repeat what I have written in another book: If I were left on a desert island, this is the one nutrient I would choose if I had only a single choice.[2]

The roster of vitamin C achievements sounds like

science fiction, but it isn't; it is fact as proved by laboratory and human tests. Vitamin C and ascorbic acid have been used successfully for the following ailments:

Cholesterol (high) and hardening of arteries
Infections
Allergies
Ulcers
Arthritis
Calcium deposits
Poor iron absorption
Gastrointestinal disorders
Barbiturate shock
Poisonous insect and snake bites
Healing from surgery
Glaucoma
Heat stroke
Low back pain
Slipped disc
Lead poisoning
Cadmium poisoning (from air and water pollution)
Liver disease
Wound healing
Atherosclerosis
Cardiovascular problems
Lockjaw
Nasal and gum bleeding
Childhood diseases
Aging
Adrenal exhaustion
Stress
Hay fever
Poison oak and ivy
Fever

Mononucleosis
Infectious hepatitis
Respiratory problems
Prickly heat rash
Diarrhea

This is not the end of the list; it is merely the beginning. Vitamin C, or ascorbic acid, is a natural antibiotic that can be used without dangerous side effects in the treatment of *any* infection. The explanation may be this: a normal, healthy body should be slightly acid (the TV antacid commercials to the contrary). Germs cannot survive easily in an acid medium, whereas they can thrive in an alkaline environment. Vitamin C is an acid medium. People who have died from infections have been found, on autopsy, to have no vitamin C at all in their bloodstream. In addition to being a natural antibiotic, ascorbic acid is also a natural diuretic, one that does not produce the insidious side effects of drug diuretics.

The lack of mental alertness in the aging may be at least partially due to a deficiency of vitamin C.[3] Dr. Roger J. Williams states that this vitamin may be a factor in delaying aging. He also reports that it has relieved low back pain, may be at least one factor for preventing cancer, and is one of the vitamins used with success in megavitamin (large amounts) therapy for schizophrenia and other types of mental illness.[4]

Vitamin C is by no means new. In 1747, James Lind, M.D., a British physician, discovered it in citrus fruit and used it as a preventive for scurvy, a plague at that time for the sailors in the British navy. But using citrus fruit as a sole source of vitamin C in 1747 is not the same thing as using it as the sole source in the 1980's. I have heard people say smugly: "Oh, I get plenty of vitamin C in my diet. I drink a glassful of orange juice every morning without fail!" (This is often a chemical combination with little vitamin C added.)

I am sorry to disillusion such people, but in these days, this amount of vitamin C is a laugh. To begin with, one glassful of natural orange juice contains approximately no more than 100 mg. of vitamin C. One cigarette uses up 25 mg., and air and water pollution, as well as stress, more than removes the rest from the body. Vitamin C is stored in your adrenal glands. Any kind of stress—a fight with your husband or wife, an emotional shock or worry about a child, overdue bills, or whatever—destroys all of the vitamin C in your adrenals in seconds! The miracles that vitamin C can accomplish are not accomplished with a drop-in-the-bucket dosage, but in massive amounts. Dr. Pauling and nutritional physicians who work constantly with vitamin C believe that the amount suggested in the Recommended Dietary Allowance by the Food and Nutrition Board of the National Academy of Science in this country is a farce. Dr. Pauling himself uses 10,000 mg. of ascorbic acid daily and has done so for thirteen years, during which time he says he has not had a single cold. This dosage is over 150 times that of the minimum dosage suggested in the Recommended Dietary Allowance.

Not only are we surrounded by environmental and emotional stresses of all kinds, but those who insist we get enough vitamin C in our foods should realize that according to a study made in Ireland, 80 percent of the vitamin C in our food is lost in cooking. Since it is a water-soluble vitamin, most of it goes into the cooking water and down the sink. Even exposure to the air can cause a loss of vitamin C in foods. And the late W. J. McCormick, M.D., of Toronto, said that of approximately 6,000 patients, he never found a smoker with a normal level of vitamin C.[5]

Unfortunately, human beings, guinea pigs and monkeys cannot synthesize their own vitamin C. Some veterinarians are now telling us that it is not wise to take a chance with sick dogs or cats, either. They are advocating vitamin C for them in high doses for infections.

How about controlling colds with vitamin C? I have received letters from readers complaining that ascorbic acid had never cured a cold in their families. I agree. I, too, have never known vitamin C to cure a cold, but I have known it to prevent a cold, and my family and I have done it time and time again. If you, like the average person, have little or no vitamin C in your bloodstream, it is too late to administer it after a cold has taken hold, although it may shorten its duration and lighten the symptoms somewhat. Dr. Pauling advises one to take 500 mg. of ascorbic acid (available in inexpensive tablets of either 250 or 500 mg. potency) at the *first* sign of a scratchy throat or other sign of a beginning cold. If you put it off, it is too late and will not abort the cold. Dr. Pauling then suggests taking another 500 mg. every few hours. He says that, even when symptoms subside, one should keep it up because the virus is still there and may reassert itself.

I, and most people I know, take not 500 mg. but 1,000 mg. every hour or so at the slightest sign of an impending cold, and it works like a charm. Don't be surprised if your kidneys overact. This is usual. Calcium used as a buffer together with vitamin C helps.

The late Fred R. Klenner, M.D. suggested a calcium tablet with every 1,000 mg. of ascorbic acid. This keeps you from becoming nervous.[6] A friend of mine who had not heard of this suggestion told me she became jittery when she took large amounts of vitamin C. I told her about the calcium trick and she had no more trouble. However, newer information decrees that the cut-off point in taking large amounts of vitamin C is the appearance of diarrhea. Again, don't be surprised if vitamin C activates your kidneys.

I agree with Dr. Pauling about not giving up too soon. I have told the story elsewhere about the first time I tried vitamin C in massive doses for a cold accompanied by a high temperature.[7] I faithfully took 1,000 mg. of vitamin C plus a calcium lactate tablet each hour and nothing happened. Later in the day, I began to feel a little better directly after taking a dose, but the feeling soon disappeared. I had started at 10 A.M. and by nightfall my temperature was still high. I had just decided the treatment wouldn't work, but took one more dose anyway. Suddenly my temperature fell to normal as if it had been cut off with a knife! Apparently that last dose was necessary to bring up the vitamin C level in my bloodstream to normal. Had I stopped sooner, the virus would have triumphed. Vitamin C has since rescued me, and the members of my family, as well as most of my friends, from so many disturbances that I would not be without it anywhere, any time, including on that desert isle. Properly used, its action is dramatic.

Dr. Klenner of North Carolina was perhaps one of the earliest physicians to have outstanding success treating his patients with vitamin C. He uses massive amounts, usually by injection, for truly serious diseases, including polio. He told of an eighteen-month-old girl who had been paralyzed by polio and became unconscious after a convulsion; she appeared to be dead, there being no heart sounds or pulse. He injected 6,000 mg. of vitamin C into her blood, and four hours later she was cheerful and alert, though paralyzed on one side. A second injection returned her to normal. All paralysis had disappeared.[8]

Dr. Klenner found that massive doses of vitamin

C can abort virus pneumonia, and save patients from fatal encephalitis related to stubborn head and chest colds. He said that it also neutralizes, possibly controls, virus production. He added: "In treatments of burns, ascorbic acid in sufficient amounts is truly a miracle substance." He recommended one or two gm. per day (1,000 to 2,000 mg.) for swift healing. He found it has primary and lasting good effects in pregnancy, too.

Dr. Klenner told a dramatic story of a man who came to him with chest pains, barely able to breathe. He claimed that something had "stung" him. Dr. Klenner immediately injected 12,000 mg. of ascorbic acid. The C neutralized the poison. Dr. Klenner sent the man home to hunt for the culprit that had stung him, and he returned with a puss caterpillar, which had raised over forty welts on his skin. Dr. Klenner said: "Except for vitamin C, this man would have died from shock and asphyxiation."[9]

The bite of a black widow spider has also yielded to vitamin C.[10]

Dr. Klenner credited vitamin C with healing corneal ulcers. Due to the flare-up of the use of an old-fashioned match by one of his patients, a corneal burn resulted. Dr. Klenner prescribed 1,000 mg. of vitamin C per hour for fifty hours. The cornea became normal in twenty-four hours. He also used ascorbic acid for ulcers, radiation sickness, rheumatic fever, scarlet fever, pancreatitis, whooping cough and TB.

Although most observers believe there is no safe therapy for pesticide poisoning, Dr. Klenner believed differently. He found vitamin C helpful if given immediately. Three boys were exposed to pesticide poisoning from a spray plane. One received little exposure and was released. He treated the second boy with massive doses of vitamin C and the boy recovered. The third boy went to another doctor who applied different treatment and the boy died.[11]

Of three children suffering from nasal diphtheria simultaneously, one was given massive doses of vitamin C and is now a graduate nurse. Both of the other children, treated elsewhere by other means, died.

One of the most startling cases of all was that of a four-year-old girl who received a snake bite on her leg. When she was brought to Dr. Klenner's office, she was crying from pain and vomiting. While Dr. Klenner waited twenty-five minutes for an antivenom skin test reaction, he gave her an injection of 4,000 mg. of vitamin C. Before the antivenom had been administered, the child had stopped crying and vomiting and was laughing and drinking a glass of orange juice. She said, "Come on, Daddy, let's go home. I'm all right now." Hourly reports by phone throughout the night showed only a slight swelling and a temperature of 99°F. A second injection of vitamin C returned her to normal. No antibiotic had been used.[12]

Irwin Stone, the mentor from whom Dr. Pauling first learned of vitamin C therapy, writes: "Fred R. Klenner, M.D., for the past quarter century pioneered the megascorbic acid theory of a wide variety of diseases. He obtained fantastically successful clinical results using up to 100 gm. or more of ascorbate a day both orally and intravenously. He recommended to his adult patients the continuous daily intake of 10 gm. or 10,000 mg.

"For children he prescribed 1 gm. (1,000 mg) of ascorbic acid a day for each year of age up to ten and then 10 gm. (10,000 mg.) daily thereafter. He reported unusual continuous good health and freedom from disease in his patients."[13]

Dr. Stone gives documented proof of the success of

vitamin C as a treatment for the illnesses listed at the beginning of this chapter. He discusses in detail the successful effect of vitamin C in such diseases as viral infections (including hepatitis, herpes, measles and chicken pox), bacterial infections (including TB, pneumonia and whooping cough), cancer and leukemia, strokes, arthritis and rheumatism, asthma, hay fever and effects of smoking, ulcers, diabetes and hypoglycemia, mental illness, poisons and toxins, bone fractures and shock. This is truly a big order. But that is not all.

Emil Ginter, M.D., of Czechoslovakia, one of the first researchers to note the good effect of vitamin C on cholesterol, has found that a *lack* of vitamin C in guinea pigs (which, like man, do not manufacture vitamin C) has led to the formation of gallstones.[14]

Other researchers have found that vitamin C is needed for the proper function of the brain and the lenses of the eyes. They have found that large amounts of vitamin C can prevent some types of cataracts in people who are susceptible to them, and can retard the growth of cataracts already beginning to form.[15]

Dr. Therese Terroine, a French researcher, has found that vitamin C can cover, at least for a time, the lack of B and other vitamins. She says: "Vitamin C plays a protective role against deficiencies of other vitamins."[16]

Two other interesting findings are that the need of vitamin C increases with age[17] and that losses of ascorbic acid are high in foods cooked in aluminum pans.[18]

Adelle Davis told how, after learning about Dr. Klenner's vitamin C therapy, she cured a case of mumps in her own son in one day. She gave him 1,000 mg. of vitamin C, plus a little calcium every hour for ten hours. By night the mumps were gone. For small children, she suggests that mothers dissolve 100 tablets of 250 mg.

potency of vitamin C, or 50 tablets of 500 mg. potency in a cup of boiling water and refrigerate. One teaspoon of this solution equals approximately 500 mg. of ascorbic acid, and can be added to juice for palatability.[19]

Now, with this impressive history of the use of vitamin C, what about the scare stories that have appeared in the press following the publication of Dr. Pauling's book, *Vitamin C and the Common Cold*?[20] Such shockers as warnings that vitamin C causes kidney stones, diabetes and other ailments have appeared. One doctor was quoted as saying that vitamin C is dangerous and one could become "hooked" on it! Are these criticisms true or false?

Dr. Klenner stated indignantly that large doses of ascorbic acid do *not* cause diabetes mellitus. He adds that the ascorbic acid-kidney stone scare is a myth. And he had probably as much or more experience with this therapy than any doctor in the world.

Dr. Abram Hoffer, who uses megavitamin therapy of niacin (B-3) and vitamin C for schizophrenia, said in a letter to a medical journal: "I have used megadoses of ascorbic acid, 3,000 to 30,000 mg. per day, since 1953 on perhaps over 1,000 patients. During this long period I have not seen one case of kidney stone formation, or miscarriage, or dehydration or of any other serious toxicity. It is my impression ... that it does reduce the frequency of colds."[21]

A physician at a veteran's hospital in the Midwest wrote the following in the magazine *Let's Live:* "In keeping with the vitamin C controversy, let me say that 3,000 mg. of vitamin C has definitely proved its effectiveness in preventing upper respiratory infection. It also prevents new bedsores and heals old ones.

"I also believe that vitamin C can bring about, as

reported elsewhere, a reversibility in the atherosclerotic process, and in so doing, it must also have a beneficial effect on the heart. No reported cases of coronary attacks or strokes have occurred [in this hospital] since vitamin C therapy was instituted."

Another physician told me confidentially that the widely publicized scare stories may well have been a result of the fact that Dr. Pauling took the drug industry to task for making useless cold remedies instead of promoting a simple, inexpensive vitamin C. He also took to task so-called tests on the common cold, stating that the report of the therapy used was not accurate nor the dosages of vitamin C sufficient.

It is true that the FDA has seized sodium ascorbate (not ascorbic acid) in some health stores. The reason is that, since the Pauling book, there has been a run on the vitamin and a shortage developed. Japan, I am told, rushed supplies of sodium ascorbate to this country to fill the gap. Because this compound contains salt (not stated on the label) and is considered unacceptable for those on low-salt diets, it was removed from the stores.

There are a few side effects from taking massive doses of ascorbic acid. Dr. Klenner noted that it may cause diarrhea in some cases. Dr. Hoffer says: "The most common side effect is diarrhea. If it does occur, one merely reduces the dose by 1 or 2 gm. (1,000 or 2,000 mg.)."[22] This may also be a sign that the high amount used is no longer necessary.

I have observed a few people who developed a rash as a result of taking massive doses of ascorbic acid. However, this has been blamed by some on the fillers used in some tablets. Many people can be allergic to almost anything. I have one friend who thrives on vitamin C injections, but breaks out in a rash on eating any kind of fruit, even that just picked fresh while she was in Hawaii.

If you wonder if you have a vitamin C deficiency, one clue, in addition to frequent colds and infections, is recurring black and blue marks, or bruises on your skin.

THE BIOFLAVONOIDS

Many people do not realize there are two kinds of vitamin C; the whole complex is called the bioflavonoids.

If you had access to a device known as "a black light" you could probably find out for yourself whether or not you are deficient in this type of vitamin C. This is how it is done: Hold up your hand, with the black light behind it, to see into the inside of the tissues of your hand. If the tissues appear to be watery, you may have this bioflavonoid deficiency. These tissues should be held together firmly with a gluelike substance called collagen.

Collagen is a protein factor in fibrous tissue. With it, the tissues appear firm and well-knit; without it they appear loose and watery. Thus, when there is a bioflavonoid deficiency, it seems logical that germs and a virus can travel by these waterways throughout the body. If, however, the collagen is strong and the tissues firmly held together, they can stop an infection from further invasion, whether it is a germ, a virus, an allergy such as hay fever, or even poison oak or ivy.

The greater the bioflavonoid deficiency, the more bioflavonoids are needed until the condition is corrected and the bulwark against such invasion becomes impregnable. The second type of vitamin C, ascorbic acid, is a quick method; the first is slower but perhaps more lasting. The quick method is by the use of ascorbic acid in massive amounts; the slower way is by use of the bioflavonoids. The latter may be preferable because it *prevents* a vitamin C deficiency.

As I have explained, ascorbic acid is only one factor in the vitamin C family or complex, usually known as the bioflavonoids. Ascorbic acid is synthetic (synthesized from corn glucose); the bioflavonoids are natural, because so far chemists have not found a way to synthesize them. However both forms of C have their values. Some people take both.

Actually, there is much confusion about the bioflavonoids because they may, or may not, be a vitamin C and are often called vitamin P. Vitamin P was isolated from oranges in 1936 by a Hungarian researcher, Albert Szent-Györgyi, who received a Nobel Prize for his work. Vitamin P was also found in red peppers, from which paprika is made. But there is an overlap between vitamin C and vitamin P. The richest source of vitamin P is rind of orange. For example, in one fresh-peeled orange containing the white membrane, there are 1,000 mg. of bioflavonoids (or vitamin P) and 60 mg. of ascorbic acid (or vitamin C). Therefore, eating the whole fruit (minus the outer skin) or drinking unstrained juice is better than drinking strained juice. The vitamin P factor is also found in lemons, grapes, plums, black currants, grapefruit, apricots, cherries and blackberries. A lesser amount is found in green leaves. Extremely high amounts are found in acerola cherries and rose hips. (The hips form after the rose has finished blooming.)

Research shows that vitamins P and C are closely related and work together. Vitamin P is derived from the vitamin C citrus fruits, especially oranges. Szent-Györgyi believes that scurvy, once thought to be due to a deficiency of vitamin C alone, is actually due to a combined deficiency of vitamins P and C (ascorbic acid).

Today, the name vitamin P has largely been dropped and the name bioflavonoids, an interrelated combination of several factors, including natural vitamin C, is used in its place. The bioflavonoids include citrin, hesperidin, quercetin and rutin. The combination of these factors plus C, under the name bioflavonoids, has been credited with some dramatic healings.

The bioflavonoids can accomplish results that vitamin C alone cannot. Their main function alone is to strengthen capillary fragility, prevent bleeding and act as a safe anti-coagulant (one without the dangerous effects of the drug anti-coagulants). Charles E. Brambel, M.D., of the Mercy Hospital of Baltimore, found the bioflavonoids safe as an anti-coagulant and administered them in 100 mg. doses, four times daily, clearing the hemorrhaging areas quickly.[23]

Part of the credit for the good effects of the bioflavonoids goes to the related factor, rutin, usually added to the bioflavonoid complex because it is so compatible with the other factors. Rutin, also a factor of vitamin P, is found most abundantly in buckwheat or eucalyptus. It is responsible for strengthening the capillary fragility in the body and thus can help prevent a stroke. In a study reported by a medical journal, high blood pressure in animals was induced. Those not fed rutin died; those given rutin did not show any signs of hemorrhaging.[24] However, rutin is not given primarily to lower blood pressure, but to strengthen the fragile capillaries.[25]

A Hungarian study showed that rats deprived of bioflavonoids for two months exhibited an abnormal increase in the permeability of their capillaries.[26]

Ailments in addition to high blood pressure, for which the bioflavonoids have been reported effective, include:

Rheumatic fever
Respiratory infections
Arthritis
Polio
Miscarriages
Hemorrhoids
Varicose veins
Tuberculosis
Gum bleeding (pink toothbrush bristles may also indicate bleeding elsewhere in the body)
Retinal hemorrhages
Radiation sickness
Rh factor
Bursitis
Arteriosclerosis (see chapter 17)
Coronary thrombosis (blood clot)
Some uterine bleeding

Catharyn Elwood gives a plethora of cases, all medically documented, of dramatic uses of the bioflavonoids.[27] One was an elderly man, a diabetic, with broken capillaries and blood oozing from his eyes. Thanks to bioflavonoids, his eye condition returned to normal in just six weeks. A nineteen-year-old boy developed serious bleeding following a tooth extraction. He was also a victim of abdominal bleeding, and resulting exploratory surgery required 200 transfusions. He was given bioflavonoids plus extra C and in ten months was found to have a normal red blood count. All bleeding, pain and swelling had ceased.

People who are plagued with bursitis and can find no relief are often told that surgery or ultrasonic therapy is their only hope. Not so. Catharyn Elwood tells the story of a man who was suffering from this ailment. With 200 mg. of bioflavonoids, prescribed by nutritional physicians to be used three times a day (a total of 600 mg. daily), the pain and swelling had almost disappeared in twenty-four hours. In seventy-two hours the disturbance had gone, leaving only a slight, reminiscent tenderness.[28]

Bioflavonoids can also protect against colds by preventing a vitamin C deficiency. One doctor told me that although he was exposed to colds from his patients throughout the winter time he never contracted one because he took two bioflavonoids three times a day (a total of six) throughout the cold season. (Bioflavonoids are not usually taken in such high doses as is ascorbic acid.)

Which form of C is best? Ascorbic acid or the bioflavonoids? My answer is: both. Bioflavonoids work more slowly to reduce the C deficiency and do what ascorbic acid cannot do—build resistance to capillary fragility. On the other hand, if you have an emergency, such as an infection or a threat of a cold, ascorbic acid in massive amounts, used quickly and often, is needed. Dr. Pauling and Irwin Stone take this vitamin by dissolving crystals of it in water and drinking it.

The average person takes ascorbic acid in tablet form, either 250 mg. or 500 mg. per tablet, because it is more convenient. These two men, who have taken massive doses of ascorbic acid for years with excellent results, could well try bioflavonoids, too. It is possible they might find they need ascorbic acid only for emergencies or following stress (which robs the adrenals of their vitamin C as explained previously). I know nutritionists who follow the same principle, taking the vitamin C complex as they take the vitamin B complex; they take both. Taking a certain amount of ascorbic acid daily, plus two or three bioflavonoids daily, is hard to beat.

The bioflavonoids are often sold under the name CPR. The "C" stands for vitamin C (ascorbic acid), the "P" for the bioflavonoids and the "R" for rutin. Read your labels for the amounts of each. Are they safe? Bicknell and Prescott state: "Substances with a vitamin P action, such as hesperidin and rutin, are virtually nontoxic even in large doses. Numbers of clinical studies show that vitamin P is an essential factor in human nutrition."[29]

REFERENCES

1. Linus Pauling. *Vitamin C and the Common Cold.* San Francisco: W. H. Freeman, 1970.

2. Linda Clark. *Get Well Naturally.* Paperback edition. New York: Arco Publishing, 1972.

3. *The Medical Journal of Australia.* May 8, 1971.

4. Roger J. Williams. *Nutrition Against Disease.* Paperback edition. New York: Bantam, 1973.

5. *Prevention.* June, 1955.

6. Adelle Davis. *Let's Eat Right to Keep Fit.* Paperback edition. New York: New American Library, 1970.

7. Linda Clark, *op. cit.*

8. Adelle Davis, *op. cit.*

9. Fred R. Klenner. "Observations on the Dose and Administration of Ascorbic Acid When Employed Beyond the Range of a Vitamin." *The Journal of Applied Nutrition.* Vol. 23, Nos. 3 and 4, 1971.

10. *Ibid.*

11. *Ibid.*

12. *Ibid.*

13. Irwin Stone. *Vitamin C: The Healing Factor.* Paperback edition. New York: Today Press (Grosset and Dunlap), 1972.

14. *The Lancet.* November 27, 1971.

15. *British Journal of Nutrition.* November, 1971.

16. *World Reviews of Nutrition and Dietetics.* Vol 2, pp. 103–130, 1960.

17. *Prevention.* June, 1972.

18. *Nutritional Abstracts and Reviews.* April, 1972. Abstract No. 3147.

19. Adelle Davis, *op. cit.*

20. Linus Pauling, *op. cit.*

21. *New England Journal of Medicine.* September 9, 1971.

22. *Ibid.*

23. J. I. Rodale and staff. *The Complete Book of Vitamins.* Emmaus, Pa.: Rodale Books, 1966.

24. *The American Heart Journal.* August, 1951.

25. Bicknell and Prescott. *The Vitamin in Medicine.* New York: Grune & Stratton, 1953.

26. *Nutritional Abstracts and Reviews.* April, 1972. Abstract No. 3153.

27. Catharyn Elwood. *Feel Like a Million.* Paperback edition. New York: Pocket Books, 1965.

28. *Ibid.*

29. Bicknell and Prescott, *op. cit.*

See also:

Norman Cousins. *Anatomy of an Illness.* New York: W. W. Norton Company, 1979.

Richard Passwater. *Cancer and Its Nutritional Therapies.* New Canaan, Conn.: Keats Publishing, 1978.

15
The Magic Minerals

Vitamins are indeed marvelous, but they still are not as marvelous as minerals—a fact that surprises most people. Charles Northen, M.D., a government consultant and one of the earliest nutritional physicians, explained the reason many years ago. He said: "It is not commonly realized that the vitamins control the body's appropriation of minerals . . . in the absence of minerals *vitamins have no function*. Lacking vitamins, the system can make use of the minerals, but lacking minerals, *the vitamins are useless*." (U.S. Senate document #264)

This means that we can get along without vitamins, perhaps, but we cannot get along without minerals. The reason for this is that the human body can manufacture some of the vitamins (the B vitamins in the intestinal tract, vitamin D from sunshine, as examples), but the body cannot manufacture its own minerals. They must be supplied by food and water. According to Bernard Spur, Ph.D., all life, whether vegetable, animal or human, depends upon minerals.[1] When they are adequately supplied, they make a strong, healthy body. When they are lacking—individually or collectively—disease sets in.

Dr. Melchior Dikkers, a retired professor of biochemistry at Loyola University, of Los Angeles, believes that mineral-starved foods threaten millions of Americans despite the country's reputation of being "the best fed nation on earth." Dr. Dikkers says: "Malnutrition exists in the U.S. but it is not caused by a lack of food, but a lack of nutrients in the food due to mineral-poor soil, chemical fertilizers, preservatives and refining processes used in food preparation."

Dr. Dikkers adds that an average 150-pound human is composed of 30 trillion cells that are dependent on proper mineral balance for normal functioning. Like Dr. Spur, he states that without these minerals, disease can set in.

Actually, we are made of minerals. A person, animal or plant is a fleshy envelope made of water, air and minerals. For instance, our bones and teeth are largely made of calcium and the red blood cells must have sufficient iron in order to prevent anemia.

In the 1930s vitamins were "discovered" and everyone became so excited about them that they forgot all about the longer known minerals. The vitamins stole the limelight from the minerals at that time and are still doing so. We may be looking frantically for health in the wrong direction. Vitamins play their part, of course; but the minerals liberate the vitamins to do their work, so they must be given first consideration in acquiring or maintaining health.

It is impossible to find a plant that carries a full vitamin content unless minerals in large amounts are also present. Nature brings minerals into the leaf veins before she can begin to manufacture vitamins.

B. A. Howard in his "Formula for a Human Body" says: "If minerals are in short supply, trouble results and health is threatened. We know that rats, guinea pigs and other animals can be made diseased, or returned to health, by controlling *the minerals only* in their food."

Why is this true? Dr. George Crile has explained that the cell is similar to an electric battery, made up, as other batteries, of positive and negative polarity. For example, the one-celled amoeba has a normal electrical potential of about 20 millivolts. If the normal voltage is reduced to zero, the amoeba begins to slow down. When this activity is slowed, the health of the cell is threatened. When the activity is stopped, and no more electrical motion is noted, the one-celled animal dies. But if an electrical current is introduced before complete cessation of movement, the cell begins to regenerate and once more becomes active and healthy. The cell is selective and will take or reject a substance according to its needs. Thus, says Dr. Crile, if we supply any cell with an electrolytic solution containing the essential chemicals and minerals, the cell can reestablish its electrical balance and return to health. This solution for cell feeding, growth and health would require the combination of an excess of all essential minerals (electrolytes) in a water base in nontoxic assimilable form, he believes.

Dr. Alexis Carrel showed this principle when he kept a heart alive and beating for years outside the body in a solution containing the proper nutrients. According to Dr. Crile, if we can do the same thing within the body— feed the cells the minerals they need to maintain their full electrical potential—then we have found the secret of health. Of course, in addition to the minerals, the body needs vitamins, fats and amino acids (from proteins), for the body is also composed of them all and they need to be constantly replaced. However, the minerals must be there first, or the other elements are not assimilated properly.

Fewer vitamins as well as proteins may be required if the mineral supply is abundant. Ragner Berg, a researcher, discovered in his experiments that if minerals were sufficiently supplied to the body in proper balance, only 25 to 30 instead of 70 gm. of protein daily were necessary. As the scientists put it, minerals have a sparing action on vitamins and protein, meaning that less are necessary. I have seen people who stayed well by taking minerals, without vitamin supplements. I have not seen anyone who remained well who took vitamins without minerals in some form.

There is a reason for this. We are told that 3 billion body cells die every minute. In good health or in youth (when the mineral supply is high), these cells are replaced as fast as they die. But during aging or illness, when the mineral supply is depleted, the cell growth slows down and reproduction finally stops, resulting in death. The person is said to have died of "natural causes" and/or "old age," whereas the cause may have been a mineral deficiency. The body does not need to die around seventy, the average age of death. Look at those who have lived far beyond the one-hundred mark during biblical days as well as in some countries today. There are many amazing cases of regeneration from adding minerals alone to the diet. Minerals may also be a means of keeping you young.

What are the necessary minerals? What is meant by the major minerals? Trace minerals?

The major minerals occur in the body, and are needed in large amounts. Calcium, phosphorus and magnesium are some examples.

Trace minerals are not called minor minerals because they are too important to be considered lesser elements.

But since they only exist in very tiny amounts, or in traces, they are known as the trace minerals. But even the trace is necessary to the proper functioning of the human body. Iodine is an example of a trace mineral. Very little of it is needed, but it is still necessary.

Here is one approximate scientific composite analysis of the body's chemical-mineral content:

ELEMENT	PERCENTAGE
Oxygen	65
Carbon	18
Hydrogen	10
Nitrogen	3
Calcium	2
Phosphorus	1.1
Potassium	0.35
Sulfur	0.25
Sodium	0.15
Chlorine	0.15
Magnesium	0.05
Iron	0.004
Manganese	0.00013
Copper	0.00015
Iodine	0.00004
Cobalt	undetermined
Zinc	undetermined

And others not yet identified.

HOW CAN EACH MINERAL BENEFIT YOU?

CALCIUM

Calcium is present in greater abundance in the body than any other mineral. It builds bones and teeth. It calms nerves, aids insomnia, helps blood clotting to be normal, and is necessary for rhythmic heart action. It also displaces the strontium 90 present in radioactive fallout.

Calcium is one of the two minerals (the other is iron) that needs acid for assimilation. If acid in some form is not present in the body, calcium is not dissolved and cannot be held in solution for distribution where it is needed. Instead, it can pile up in tissues or joints as calcium deposits, leading to such disturbances as arthritis, bursitis and related diseases.

How do these deposits occur? Much the same way that the lining builds up in a teakettle. When the water is hard (which is good, since hardness denotes a higher ratio of minerals than soft water contains) but lacks the right pH or acidity, the minerals cannot be dissolved on the lining of the teakettle any more than in the human body. If you try to scrub off these deposits in the teakettle or even from the inside of a water distiller, you will find it is almost impossible to remove them. But if you put some apple cider vinegar into the teakettle with some water to cover, and let stand overnight, you will find the deposit dissolved and loosened for easy removal. Dr. deForest C. Jarvis, who wrote of Vermont folk medicine, gave apple cider vinegar to cattle with their feed rations. As a result, their arthritic symptoms disappeared. According to Dr. Jarvis, the human body can also use, with good results, some of this vinegar solution added to the drinking water. Another form of acid, vitamin C, together with calcium, was recommended by Adelle Davis for arthritis. A lack of hydrochloric acid can be a factor in the lack of assimilation of calcium, iron and protein.

Calcium also needs vitamin D for proper assimilation.

What are the results of calcium deficiency?

The improper assimilation of calcium, or a deficiency of it, causes tooth decay, soft bones, rickets, nervousness and irritability, insomnia, cramps (especially in the legs), heart palpitation and even convulsions.

What kind of calcium is best?

No one kind of calcium is best for everyone; also, different kinds of calcium may do different things. For example, calcium lactate seems to be quickly and easily assimilated and is a favorite as an aid for insomnia. Calcium *lactate* differs from calcium *gluconate* only in that a different acid is used to process the calcium for easier assimilation.

Bone meal is an especially important kind of calcium for several reasons. Medical textbooks tell us that approximately 99 percent of the calcium in our bodies is in the bones, with the remaining 1 percent in the blood which is ready to distribute it to tissues or nerves, wherever needed. If, however, we are not getting enough calcium, the body becomes frantic and begins to borrow, on a Peter-to-pay-Paul basis. Two Cornell University researchers, Dr. Lennart Krook and Dr. Leo Lutwalk, state that the bones do not lose calcium evenly. All the bones are asked to give up their valuable calcium supply when a deficiency occurs, but, according to these researchers, the jaw bone, in which the teeth are rooted, shows the greatest loss, resulting in inflamed and bleeding gums. When 1,000 mg. of calcium (calcium gluconate and calcium carbonate) were given patients daily for six months, X rays proved that *fresh bone had appeared.*[2]

Other studies have revealed that bone meal has arrested cavities, or in some cases has filled or repaired them naturally. Bone meal has also been shown[3] to speed healing of fractures, since bone, an ingredient of bone meal, seems to help bone repair. Oldsters who take bone meal on a regular basis[4] have been found to have fewer fractures. As people grow older, they tend to assimilate calcium less easily from milk and food sources, possibly because of a decline of hydrochloric acid. Taking an easily assimilated form of calcium and/or bone meal plus acid provides them with an adequate supply of this mineral.

The Swedish people are turning to bone meal to prevent tooth decay.

Dr. Alfred Aslander, of Sweden, internationally known for his research on tooth decay and how to prevent it, warns that one type of bone meal is dangerous. This type is known as *bone ash*, manufactured by a cheap process of igniting bones and destroying the organic matter. It releases a form of fluorine that has poisoned cattle. Dr. Aslander says it should *never* be used for animals or human beings. It can be recognized in supplement form by its chalk-white color, and no taste or odor. True bone meal, on the other hand, contains organic matter plus small amounts of trace minerals. It is slightly yellow in color with a faint animal taste and odor.

The label on my jar of bone meal tablets, purchased from a health store, states that it contains natural vitamin D, calcium and phosphorus in the correct ratio, plus various trace minerals and red bone marrow.

Food sources of calcium include milk (and milk products such as yogurt, kefir and cheese), whole grains and unrefined cereals.

PHOSPHORUS

Phosphorus works in combination with calcium, but occurs in more foods, including proteins, so that there is rarely a shortage of it in the diet. However, when phosphorus is excreted from the body, it takes calcium with it;

so if the phosphorus content is high, and calcium is not raised to balance it, a calcium deficiency can result. There should be a ratio of 2.5 calcium to 1 phosphorus. Because most people get enough phosphorus in their diet, and need more calcium, not phosphorus, some calcium supplements are available that do not include phosphorus. Lecithin and brewer's yeast, as well as meat, are especially high in phosphorus, and *extra calcium should be added to compensate*. A practical method of adding it to brewer's yeast is to add to every pound of the yeast one-fourth cup of powdered calcium lactate or one-half cup of calcium gluconate (which occurs in a coarser form) and mix thoroughly. By premixing, it will be ready to use as needed.

Leg cramps often occur when too much phosphorus is taken, even when calcium is added to the diet. The remedy is simple: merely step up the intake of calcium to correct the imbalance.

MAGNESIUM

Magnesium is one of our newer minerals, at least as far as understanding its benefits is concerned. It is of tremendous importance. Most people are deficient in it. Like calcium, it displaces the strontium 90 present in radioactive fallout. It has also been found to protect against and reverse kidney stones; has been used to treat severe angina and coronary thrombosis; has been used successfully for prostate troubles; has dramatically arrested polio; has been found helpful for alcoholics (alcohol destroys magnesium in the body); has been used to disperse irritability, depression and disagreeable behavior displayed by heavy drinkers; has been used to treat mental and emotional problems such as irrational and confused states

and even convulsions and insanity. It seems to be a specific in the treatment of neuromuscular disorders, nervousness, tantrums, rages, sensitivity to noise, epilepsy
and hand tremor.[5] One test showed a man's signature
that was completely illegible. Four hours after the administration of magnesium, the handwriting was more legible
and remained so for twenty-eight hours. Then, when
magnesium was resumed, the handwriting became still
more clear and legible, and had remained so when the
man was re-tested nine days later.[6]

Magnesium and calcium carbonate are antacids and
should be taken *between* meals. Many doctors are opposed
to the use of dolomite, a combination of magnesium and
calcium. Magnesium is an antacid; calcium needs acid for
assimilation. So it seems illogical for some people to take
them both at once, for fear of cancelling the calcium
assimilation. Ralph Pressman, Ph.D., has stated: "Dolomite is a type of rock that is ground into a powder . .
the fact is overlooked that ground rock is not readily
soluble in the stomach unless there is a normal supply of
gastric juice."[7] Other researchers believe that various combined minerals in ground rock can become impacted in
the colon unless accompanied by natural plant enzymes
to break them down into soluble form.

Foods rich in magnesium are nuts, whole grain products, dry beans and peas, dark green vegetables. Soy
products are rich in magnesium. It is also found in sea
water. Cooking and food processing remove magnesium
This mineral is also available in supplement form of various types.

There is one caution to observe in connection with
magnesium. Kidneys help to regulate magnesium and
this can help or retard normal water storage in the body.
Fluorides have a strong attraction for magnesium and

can tie up this element in the cells. Thus, since those with kidney disease are also subject to danger from fluorides, this raises the question of the wisdom of drinking fluoridated water.[8]

FLUORIDES

There are two types of fluorides. The type added to drinking water in city reservoirs is *sodium* fluoride, a by-product of some fifty different types of industries, including the manufacture of phosphate fertilizers, aluminum and steel. There is a great surplus of this sodium fluoride by-product, and the industries are anxious to dispose of it. Sodium fluoride has been identified as a poison, and calcium is an antidote for fluoride poisoning.

Sodium fluoride is not the same as that found in nature, which is *calcium* fluoride. Thus, calcium fluoride is a natural source of fluoride. Dr. John Polya, eminent professor of chemistry at the University of Tasmania, says: "There are organic fluorides that are less toxic than inorganic fluorides."[9] Those who are concerned about the homeopathic cell salt calcium fluorica, to be discussed later, will be relieved to know that this source of fluoride is not dangerous.

SODIUM

According to the late John J. Miller, Ph.D.: "Sodium seems to be the conductor of the electric currents inside the body's nerve cells."[10]

Sodium is misunderstood by many people. Because so much has been said about low sodium diets, many people avoid sodium (salt). Yet it relaxes muscles. One physician, instead of restricting the use of salt by his heart patients, recommends that they dissolve liberal amounts of *sea salt or whole salt* (containing all the minerals including sodium) in water and sip when heart symptoms harass them. Whereas potassium exists in the body *cells,* sodium exists in the body *fluids* and acts to establish a balance in the electrolyte cell function. Together with potassium, it helps the correct balance of water to be retained in the body for health. Sodium can be lost through extreme sweating, resulting in leg and abdominal cramps. Sodium, in *whole* sea salt not in sodium chloride, which is ordinary table salt, and one factor only of whole salt, if taken with the other minerals is not to be feared but respected. It is crucial to good health. It has been found related to the adrenal glands. The heart requires a ratio of 100 parts sodium, 4 parts potassium and 2 parts calcium in the bloodstream.[11] Sodium is also needed by the body for the manufacture of hydrochloric acid.

POTASSIUM

Potassium is a must. It contributes to the electrical potential of the cell and aids heart rhythm. It works with sodium to maintain a balance of water in the system, thus *preventing* edema. A lack of it can cause an upset of the entire nervous system, heart seizures, weak muscular control and constipation. Potassium is found in raw foods, green leaves, blackstrap molasses and sunflower seeds.[12]

One heart specialist, Dr. Demetrio Sodi-Pallares, of Mexico, has stated that he has given up digitalis, diuretic drugs and even vasodilator agents in the treatment of various types of heart failure in preference to a low-sodium, high-potassium diet, which he has found extremely successful.[13]

Potassium provides other benefits, too. Blood pressure and gland function are dependent on sufficient potassium. As we said above,[14] nerve and muscular weakness are also involved. Dr. W. D. Snively, Jr., and Dr. R. L. Westerman write: "Probably the most common symptom of potassium deficiency is malaise, often expressed as 'not feeling well.' Muscular weakness is almost always noted and should lead one to suspect a potassium deficit."[15]

Dr. Cowan and Dr. Judge, of Scotland, found that a weakening of muscles in elderly people is common. These doctors found that "an adequate amount of potassium given to depleted people restores strength significantly."[16]

Aging or a poor diet are not the only causes of potassium deficiency. Stress, both mental and physical, can lead to a loss of potassium.

IODINE

Iodine occurs in traces only, yet it is necessary in minute amounts. It stimulates energy (though too much can cause nervousness). Most people over forty are considered deficient in iodine. Iodine contributes to the health of the thyroid gland. An iodine deficiency can cause goiter, anemia, listlessness, lack of energy, slow pulse and low blood pressure, and weight gain. The amount found in a complete mineral source of natural origin is probably sufficient for average needs.

IRON

As you already know, iron is necessary for the manufacture of good red blood cells, an abundance of energy, pink cheeks and lips, brightness of eye and a zest for living. A lack of iron causes anemia and the reverse of the above signs of health.

The symptoms of iron deficiency include weakness, fatigue, shortness of breath after exertion, heart palpitations, deformation of nails plus ridging and brittleness, headaches and lethargy.

A biochemistry textbook states: "Unlike other inorganic constituents of the body, very little iron is absorbed by the adult . . . most of the iron is ingested with the food and is eliminated with the feces. Thus the iron that remains in the body must be used over and over again."[17]

Bernard A. Bellew, M.D., says: "Excesses of absorbed iron will be stored in various organs such as the liver, bones (marrow), spleen, lungs, pancreas, skin and others. . . . There is no question that excesses of inorganic medicinal iron, as used in enrichment and fortification of foods, can lead to chronic disabling and fatal disease in some people."[18]

This statement explains why many nutritionists strenuously object to iron-fortified flour that ends up in bread, rolls, cookies, pastas and breaded foods. Iron is also added to cereals.

Anemia is not due to lack of iron alone. It can be due to a shortage of vitamins E or C, B-6, folic acid, B-12, magnesium, iodine or protein. And it can be caused by insecticides, drugs or radiation therapy.

Adelle Davis was violently opposed to the use of iron salts in the form of ferrous chloride or ferrous sulfate, especially since the latter causes so many deaths in children. She stated that the least toxic of all the iron salts are ferrous gluconate and ferrous fumarate, although the best and safest sources of iron are, of course, meats, eggs, wholegrain (unrefined and unenriched) breads and cereals, fruits and vegetables, brewer's yeast, wheat germ, and liver and blackstrap molasses.[19]

Many forms of iron are not well assimilated. Some

vitamins, including C and E, help assimilation, and sufficient hydrochloric acid in the stomach is absolutely necessary for its absorption.

MANGANESE

Many people have never heard of manganese, yet without it we could not manage to have perfect health. A deficiency has been found linked with pancreas disturbance and diabetes. Tests of 122 diabetics of all ages have proved manganese extremely low in every case.[20]

There is a search for the cause and cure of myasthenia gravis and multiple sclerosis. It appears that a lack of manganese may be a factor in both illnesses. Myasthenia gravis is a failure of muscular coordination and loss of muscle strength. Emanuel Josephson, M.D., gave his patients suffering from myasthenia gravis a diet high in protein, vitamin E, all the B vitamins and (for a limited time) 50 mg. of manganese at each meal. Relief was obtained within several weeks and remarkable recoveries were reported by Dr. Josephson.[21]

Multiple sclerosis seems to be related to the breakdown of the myelin sheath that protects the nerves. The symptoms include jerkiness, lack of coordination, staggering when walking and tremors. As in myasthenia gravis, loss of muscular control is evident. A lack of manganese is at least one factor in the disturbance.

To treat a fellow physician suffering from multiple sclerosis, Dr. Robert M. Hill, former professor of biochemistry at the University of Colorado Medical Center, recommended the use of a food high in manganese. The food used was buckwheat, rich in manganese, and it halted the progress of multiple sclerosis.[22] The symptoms disappeared and never returned. Of course one case does not prove a fact, as Dr. Hill has admitted. But he has witnessed the reversal of multiple sclerosis symptoms in animals by the use of manganese sulfate. Other laboratory studies seem to confirm his findings that a manganese deficiency may be at least one factor in the mysterious disease.

Foods high in manganese include: egg yolks, sunflower seeds, wheat germ, wholegrain cereals and flour (such as whole wheat, oatmeal, rye and buckwheat), dried peas and beans and bone meal. (Milk and milk products are low in manganese.) Also, brewer's yeast is a good source of this mineral. Manganese occurs in green leaves, if raised on good soil; but, like iron, it is not always easily assimilated.

One good source of buckwheat is buckwheat groats, which can be used as a substitute for rice. It is common in many European countries and is available in American health stores. Cooked quickly with a small amount of liquid and served with butter and whole sea salt, it is perhaps more appetizing than the long-used buckwheat flapjacks.

Manganese is also available in homeopathic form.

ZINC

Zinc is creating more and more attention. Zinc is concentrated in hair, fingernails, toenails and all parts of the nervous system, as well as in skin, liver, bones, blood, pancreas, kidneys and pituitary glands, and in the male reproductive fluid. Its use exerts a normalizing effect upon the prostate. Its lack can lead to testicular atrophy and prostate trouble. A zinc deficiency can also cause leg ulcers and leg claudication (restriction of blood flow). When sufficient in the body, zinc appears to increase blood volume in areas where blood vessels are constricted and to protect against TB chronic infections.

Wounds heal three times faster and burns are helped by added zinc. It is said that zinc may act as an antidote for some types of drug poisoning such as marijuana and hashish.

It is true that many people have become ill from getting too much zinc by contamination of air, or water from galvanized pipes or food cooked in galvanized containers. For the most part, however, zinc is considered nontoxic. The late Henry A. Schroeder, M.D., of Dartmouth Medical School, perhaps the world's outstanding specialist on trace minerals, believed that elderly people should take at least 10 mg. of zinc daily. Women who are pregnant, or take "The Pill" need zinc since they can be greatly deficient in this mineral.[23]

Zinc is playing more and more roles in health, scientists are learning. Zinc *depletion* retards learning processes in animals and humans, and is a factor in schizophrenia. Its lack is also a factor in increased fatigue, susceptibility to infection and injury, and a slowdown in alertness and scholastic achievement. If there is a zinc deficiency in the human aorta, there may be an increase of atherosclerosis.[24]

A German study showed that a zinc deficiency in growing rats caused diarrhea, growth retardation, apathy, a coat of rough hair, emaciation, skin lesions and a stilted gait. Some rats died. In those supplied with zinc after deprivation, all symptoms were completely reversed.[25] The zinc level in diabetics tends to be low. When zinc is added to the diet, vitamin A is also needed in higher amounts. And as calcium is increased, the need for zinc is proportionately increased.

An acid soil is needed to help plants extract zinc.

Whether acid is needed by the body for the same purpose is not yet known. Protein foods are much higher in zinc; carbohydrate foods, much lower.

Foods rich in zinc include brewer's yeast, bone meal, beans, nuts and seeds (especially pumpkin and sunflower seeds), wheat germ, fertile eggs, fish and meat, with liver a particularly rich source.

CHROMIUM

Chromium is another little-known mineral that can be involved with our well-being. For one thing, it helps to utilize carbohydrates and may help in some cases with glucose intolerance or low blood sugar (hypoglycemia).

At least, supplements of chromium added to the diet have restored normal glucose utilization in some diabetics as well as in others, ranging from children, through middle age to the elderly, all of whom were found to have a chromium deficiency.[26] In fact, Dr. Walter Mertz, former Chief of the Department of Biological Chemistry at Walter Reed Army Institute of Research, believes that chromium, a recently noted "micronutrient," is essential in human nutrition. He states that it plays an important role in the liver synthesis of fatty acids and cholesterol; and he raises the question, after observing tests on experimental animals, if chromium deficiency might be a factor or cause of diabetes.[27] He also believes that adding some brewer's yeast to the diet may help to prevent an impairment of glucose metabolism.

A clinical study showed that chromium, given as an oral supplement, improved glucose tolerance in four out of six diabetics.[28] In another study of a group of hospitalized children in Israel, one oral dose of chromium was given to each child. Hyperglycemia (high blood sugar) and hypoglycemia (low blood sugar) disappeared overnight. Investigators learned that the children had been drinking water with little or no chromium, and had shown the symptoms of both these disturbances prior to the chromium supplementation, which in their case brought instant results.[29]

Chromium is lost in the refining of foods. Unsaturated fats (such as corn oil), meats and whole grains are rich in the mineral. Brewer's yeast contains the highest amount. A high amount is present in bone meal, and liver, fresh or desiccated.

LITHIUM

I have received many inquiries about lithium. One woman wrote me that a friend, suffering from deep depression, had recovered in one short month as a result of lithium therapy. She wanted to know where she could get some and in what foods it occurred. My answers to both of these questions were: "I don't know." But I will share with you what little I have learned about lithium to help give you a clue to both questions. This mineral, too, is in the early discovery stage.

The excitement about lithium may have started with a 1972 report by the U.S. Public Health Service that lithium was found in the water of El Paso, Texas, whereas there was none found in the water of Dallas. The rate of commitments to mental hospitals in Dallas was six times greater than in El Paso, according to a study by Dr. Earl B. Dawson of the University of Texas Medical School at Galveston.[30]

A subsequent report appeared, stating: "The best treatment for mental disorder may be a simple, inexpensive salt derived from lithium, a common metal. Researchers at the Royal College of Psychiatrists in London have found lithium salt to be more effective for manic and depressive illness than conventional tranquilizers."[31]

Still later, *Newsweek* reported: "At least one old medication has been rediscovered: it is lithium salts, a fairly common constituent of the mineral waters dispensed at various spas around the world. Just how lithium works is unclear, but it is being used increasingly as a specific treatment for manic highs."[32] Lithium carbonate is the type reported by *Newsweek* to be in present usage.

However, doctors who are using lithium in *drug* form (methysergide) report that the consequences or aftermath are worse than the original disturbance. Patients can become suicidal after the effect of the drug has worn off and are worse than before. Even discontinuing the drug does not help. One psychiatrist warns that patients given this drug should be kept under constant supervision.[33] Even the trace mineral, lithium, can be toxic.[34]

No foods I could find contain lithium in natural form. Sea salt, providing it is *whole* sea salt, or sea water, is a safe source; a search is needed to find lithium springs in the United States as well as in Europe.

The only other help I can provide is that a presumably safe form of lithium carbonate is available in homeopathic form and could be provided by a homeopathic physician.

Lithium is known to conserve iodine and to help raise the potassium level in the body. But except for getting it naturally in your drinking water or in sea salt or homeopathically, handle with care.

OTHER MINERALS TO WATCH

There are other minerals, less well known, many of

them trace minerals but necessary just the same. An entire book could be written on minerals but I will mention these lesser known minerals briefly:

SELENIUM can act like vitamin E and prevent multiple sclerosis in poultry. But only a *minute* amount is needed. In larger amounts, it is extremely toxic to people.[35] Many researchers warn not to take selenium separately. It occurs safely in trace amounts in sea water or in natural mineral combinations (see next chapter). Some investigators conclude that selenium is a two-edged sword, meaning both good and bad.[36] An outstanding, well-known and respected nutritionist has warned, "The margin between selenium effectiveness and toxicity is very narrow."[37]

CHLORINE used continuously in our water supply, according to Joseph M. Price, M.D., is a hazard to heart function.[38] On the other hand, small amounts of chlorine help establish electrolytic balance in body cells and aid in the manufacture of hydrochloric acid.

COBALT is needed *in small amounts only* to help assimilate vitamin B-12.

COPPER helps iron to build red blood cells, and thus helps to prevent anemia. It is found in body cells. Copper deficiency has been produced by feeding rats condensed milk for extended periods. But too much copper can be toxic, whether from an intake of water standing in copper pipes, or from a surplus in the diet. Copper cooking utensils destroy vitamin C in foods on contact.

MOLYBDENUM is an antagonist to copper. A deficiency can cause uric acid formation and increased tooth decay. It is a "coming" mineral of increasing importance. Watch it!

REFERENCES

1. Bernard Spur. "Mineral Metabolism and Its Function in Nutrition." *Health Today*. Vol. 1, No. 2, 1971.

2. *Prevention*. September, 1972.

3. Linda Clark. *Stay Young Longer*. Paperback edition. New York: Pyramid Communications, 1968.

4. *Ibid.*

5. Linda Clark. "The Magic Mineral, Magnesium.' *Get Well Naturally*. Paperback edition. New York: Arco Publishing, 1972.

6. *Journal of the American Medical Association*. April 21, 1956.

7. Ralph Pressman. "Calcium, the Neglected Mineral." *National Health Federation Bulletin*. May, 1970.

8. *Clinical Physiology*. Spring, 1964.

9. John Polya. *Are We Safe?* Australia: Chester Press.

10. *The Miller Message*. Newsletter. August, 1972. (To obtain, write P.O. Box 299, West Chicago, Illinois 60185.)

11. R. H. Follis, et al. *American Journal of Pathology*. Vol. 18, p. 29, 1942.

12. *Ibid.*

13. *Prevention*. October, 1972, pp. 47–48.

14. *Ibid.*

15. *Minnesota Medicine*. June, 1965.

16. *Journal of the American Medical Association*. October 6, 1969.

17. Benjamin Harrow and Abraham Mazur. *Textbook of Biochemistry*. Seventh edition. Philadelphia: W. B. Saunders, 1958.

18. Bernard A. Bellew and Joeva Galaz Bellew. "Are We Being Overfortified with Iron?" *Let's Live*. March, 1972.

19. Adelle Davis. *Let's Get Well.* Paperback edition. New York: New American Library, 1972.

20. *Klin. Med.* Vol. 42, p. 113, 1964.

21. Emanuel Josephson. *The Thymus, Manganese and Myasthenia Gravis.* Chedney Press, 1961.

22. J. I. Rodale and staff. *The Complete Book of Minerals for Health.* Emmaus, Pa.: Rodale Press, 1972.

23. Henry A. Schroeder. *Pollution, Profits and Progress.* Brattleboro, Vt.: Stephen Greene Press, 1971.

24. *The Miller Message, op. cit.*

25. *Nutrition Abstracts and Reviews.* April, 1972. Abstract No. 3602.

26. Ruth Winter. "Mini-Metals; They Can Save Your Life or Kill You." *Science Digest.* June, 1972.

27. *Food and Nutrition.* December, 1966.

28. *Science.* May 27, 1966.

29. J. I. Rodale, *op. cit.*

30. *Organic Consumer Bulletin.* September 12, 1972.

31. *Ibid.* October 31, 1972.

32. *Newsweek.* January 8, 1973.

33. The *Lancet.* February 22, 1969.

34. J. I. Rodale, *op. cit.*

35. Erwin Di Cyan. *Vitamin E and Aging.* New York: Pyramid Communications, 1972.

36. Robert M. Downs, M.D. and J.J. Challem. "Primer of Minerals." *Let's Live.* March 1979.

37. *Prevention.* December 1979, p. 42.

38. Joseph M. Price, *Coronaries, Cholesterol, Chlorine.* New York: Pyramid Communications, 1971.

See also:

Carl C. Pfeiffer. *Zinc and Other Micro-Nutrients.* New Canaan, Conn.: Keats Publishing, 1978.

16
Where to Find Safe Sources of All Minerals

What is the best way to get your mineral supply? There are several good sources. One is from sea water, sea plants such as kelp, or whole sea salt. Charles B. Ahlson, the late expert on the value of sea water, wrote: "Remember, all minerals are in sea water in almost direct proportion to the mineral content of our bloodstream."[1]

Sam Roberts, M.D., uses alfalfa for himself and his patients, because the roots penetrate as deeply as twenty or more feet and gather an excellent mineral balance. He also uses kelp for his patients and himself because seafoods and sea plants feed upon and absorb the minerals from ocean water, thus including every mineral the body needs.

Although kelp has long been acknowledged as a source of all minerals, alfalfa, the source of many, has been overlooked. According to the late Frank Lachle, a chemical engineer: "Alfalfa has the greatest variety and largest amount of nutrients of any known plant. It is the richest food in seven vitamins and six minerals. It is the best

known source of vitamins C, B-6, D, E, K, U and betaine.
It is the best known source of the minerals calcium, iron,
magnesium, potassium sulphur and manganese, and is
high in trace minerals."

I use either of two natural mineral combination
powders—Minerals 74 available at health stores, or
Azomite, available through Rollin J. Anderson, Azome
Utah Mining Co., Sterling, Utah 64665.

SALT

Salt can provide minerals but should be chosen with
care. Most salt is not whole sea salt containing all the
minerals. Instead, it usually contains sodium chloride only.
As you have seen in the last chapter, sodium can cause
water retention in the body. Potassium can eliminate it
from the body. In sodium chloride only, the potassium
is missing. In whole sea salt, the potassium is present
and can regulate the sodium so as to drain off the
excess water. There are, of course, other minerals, too, in
whole sea salt. Some salt is sold as sea salt, and is not
whole sea salt. It originally came from the sea, yes, but in
the processing, the other minerals were leached away and
only the sodium chloride remains. Labels should be required to state whether the salt is whole or merely contains the single factor: sodium chloride. There are very
few whole sea salts available. The government has banned
them because they are not pure white, but slightly colored because of the trace minerals. A whole, natural sea
salt imported from France or Belgium was available at
many health stores. If you cannot get a whole sea salt,
then there are one or two salts that are next best: those
mined from salt mines on land. They are nearly as high
in all minerals and have been found to supply all the

minerals necessary for health. Salt dehydrated from small inland seas may be contaminated.

SEAWEEDS

Kelp and other seaweeds are among our best sources of all minerals. Seaweeds are able to convert inorganic elements into organic elements by the process of photosynthesis. Pure, unadulterated kelp, harvested from the sea, provides a rich vegetable source of all essential minerals and trace elements, plus some vitamins and protein. An analysis of kelp reveals that it includes the minerals: iodine, cobalt, manganese, iron, copper, sulphur, silicon, boron, aluminum, strontium, nickel, chromium, chlorine, potassium, magnesium, calcium, phosphorus, barium, titanium, gallium, bismuth, tin, vanadium, silver, molybdenum, zirconium, zinc and others. (Don't worry about these: they are in small traces only, and in organic form.) It also includes vitamin A, and the B vitamins, B-1, B-2, B-3, pantothenic acid and choline, as well as amino acids (protein factors).

If none of the naturally present iodine is removed from our dried kelp, one small tablet should supply you with as much iodine as found in 70 pounds of fresh vegetables and fruits; or 56 pounds of cereal grains and nuts; or 12 pounds of eggs; or almost 2 pounds of fish. Kelp contains 22 minerals plus added trace elements.[2]

Meanwhile, Jacques Ménètrier, M.D., of Switzerland, states that trace element therapy by the use of seaweeds has given good results in high blood pressure, allergies, premature aging, resistance to TB and flu. Melchior T. Dikkers states that seaweeds have antibiotic qualities, help relieve constipation and intestinal as well as respiratory irritations. They have been used for hundreds of years for diarrhea. T. J. Lyel, M.D., adds that, though the action of seaweed is slow, it can help mucous membranes, weight loss, gout, rheumatism and dropsy. It was found by researchers of McGill University in Canada to remove body radioactivity.

Probably one of the most dramatic studies of using seaweed or kelp tablets with people was done many years ago by George L. Siefert, M.D., and H. Curtis Wood, M.D., both of Philadelphia. They used Pacific Ocean kelp (Macrocystis pyrifera), presumably complete with iodine, in tablet form for their patients. They found that in 400 pregnant women placed on three kelp tablets daily, the blood count (hemoglobin) rose from 65 to 83 percent. The doctors also noted the following improvements:

Better color and quality of hair
Less brittle fingernails
Less bruising due to fragile capillaries
Relief in some types of skin problems
Definite improvement in arthritis
Relief in cases of such eye disturbances as iritis and cataracts
Less constipation
Increased sense of well-being

BREWER'S YEAST

Another source of minerals, plus added factors, is brewer's yeast. It contains at least nine B vitamins (probably more), sixteen amino acids and it contains these minerals: calcium, phosphorus, potassium, magnesium, silicon, copper, manganese, chromium, zinc, aluminum, sodium, iron, tin, boron, gold and silver. Some of these minerals may appear to be no-no's but are not to be feared because they occur in organic form and may assist the assimilation of the other minerals.

CELL SALTS

Another little known source of minerals is the homeopathic cell salts. They represent the important minerals found in the body, which should be constantly replaced to prevent a deficiency of any or all of them, so that poor health can be prevented and good health can be maintained.

Cell salts are not drugs. They are tiny, sweet-tasting, white tablets about twice as thick as the head of a pin. They contain minerals that, on analysis, have been found already to exist in the body. They are considered necessary for proper growth and maintenance of health. For this reason they are known as biochemical cell salts, or the Schuessler cell salts, named after the physician who "discovered" them. There are twelve cell salts. They have the following names, but are usually called by their abbreviations:

1. *Calcarea Phosphorica* (phosphate of lime); abbreviated as Calc. Phos.

2. *Kali Phosphoricum* (phosphate of potash or potassium), Kali. Phos.

3. *Magnesia Phosphorica* (magnesium phosphate), Mag. Phos.

4. *Natrum Phosphoricum* (phosphate of soda), Nat. Phos.

5. *Ferrum Phosphoricum* (phosphate of iron), Fer. Phos.

6. *Natrum Sulphuricum* (sulphate of soda), Nat. Sulph.

7. *Kali Sulphuricum* (sulphate of potash), Kali. Sulph.

8. *Calcarea Sulphurica* (sulphate of lime), Calc. Sulph.

9. *Kali Muriaticum* (chloride of potash), Kali. Mur.
10. *Natrum Muriaticum* (sodium chloride), Nat. Mur.
11. *Calcium Fluorica* (fluoride of lime), Calc. Fluor.
12. *Silicea* (silica).

These cell salts are not new, but merely ignored or forgotten in favor of drugs. They were discovered as early as 1873 by W. H. Schuessler, M.D. He analyzed human blood and isolated these important minerals, which are always found in human ashes after death, proving they are an integral part of the body. In countless experiments, Dr. Schuessler learned that if any of the body cells become deficient in these minerals, the deficiency causes an abnormal or diseased condition. He ascertained by noting various symptoms which minerals were lacking in his patients, and supplied them. He found that if diseases are curable at all, and the proper cell salt is chosen and given in the proper amount, the deficiency that causes the abnormality is corrected, and the body heals itself. Thus the cell salts are not used to cure anything; they are merely supplied to the body to remedy a deficiency so that health can return to the cells, and thus to the body, which is made up of cells.[3]

Mira Louise, the late Australian naturopath and nutritionist, who was a cell salt specialist, stated in her writings: "The action of these cell salts is little short of miraculous."

HOW CELL SALTS WORK

Like all homeopathic remedies cell salts may be more effective in some cases than in others because they are reduced to an almost infinitesimal degree of fineness, a process called trituration. The first trituration is made by mixing one part of the mineral with nine parts of milk sugar, pounded in a mortar for two hours. This is called the "1x" potency. When one part of the 1x potency is mixed with 9 parts of milk sugar and pulverized in the same way, it becomes the 2x potency and so on. Homeopathic potencies can reach the 200th potency or higher, which reduces the particles to almost unbelievable fineness. The cells of the body can accept and assimilate these fine particles, whereas they may reject or be unable to assimilate vitamins, which are in grosser form. Since the cell salts are absorbed by the capillaries, they must be finer than capillaries. However, both vitamins and cell salts are necessary.

HOW TO TAKE CELL SALTS

Cell salts are not dependent on the usual method of digestion, so they are not washed down with water. They are assimilated by the body by osmosis, preferably via the saliva. Thus, they should be dissolved on the tongue, or dissolved in warm water and sipped slowly. The experts tell us that they should be taken in the 3x potency, except for Calc. Fluor., Nat. Mur. and Silicea, which should be in the 6x potency.

Cell salts come in two general forms: individually or as a combination of all twelve cell salts. The combination is usually taken for the prevention of a deficiency of any or all of the cell salts, or for the maintenance of health, once you have corrected a deficiency. The individual cell salts, as described on the label, are taken in the amount of twenty-four tablets (six, four times daily). The all-in-one can be taken in the same way: but many of us, for the sake of convenience, take a small amount of the twenty-four all at once (remember that they are very tiny) or approximately a teaspoonful each morning. On reading the articles and books related to cell salts (see references, this chapter), you may decide you need one or more separate cell salts to correct a certain deficiency (for example, silicea for hair and nails). You may combine this cell salt with the all-in-one, taking it until the signs of deficiency of that cell salt disappear. Any individual cell salt may be taken between meals, or at bedtime, dissolved dry on the tongue. If you choose more than one to add to your daily intake of the all-in-one, they can be taken alternately.

When I asked a professional expert if there were any danger in taking cell salts, he said: "Absolutely not! In agricultural chemistry we add the element most lacking in the soil, as a fertilizer to the soil. The plant picks up the element and recovers. The same law applies to the biochemic theory of the biochemic cell salts. If the reservoir of the human cell is already filled, there is no danger from taking the element since the cell will merely reject it and it will be excreted from the body. Remember, cell salts are not drugs, but substances found in nature."

Cell salts are surprisingly inexpensive. In Great Britain, they are routinely stocked by health stores. In the United States, they may now be found at many health stores, but are mainly available at homeopathic pharmacies. If you do not find a source in your area, write for information to Standard Homeopathic Pharmacy, P.O. Box 21067, Los Angeles, California 90061. The homeopathic pharmacies also carry several other separate minerals such as chromium, manganese, lithium carbonate, iodine and zinc. Because of their minute potencies, they are considered safe; however, except for the all-in-one cell salt combination, homeopathic substances are not taken day-in and day-out like other minerals or vitamins. They are taken only to correct a deficiency, or a condition. In some cases of disease, only one dose of a specially prescribed homeopathic substance is sufficient. A homeopathic physician can prescribe these special remedies for you. To get the name of a homeopathic doctor near you, write to the National Center for Homeopathy, 7297 Lee Highway, Falls Church, Virginia 22402.

The cell salts are a do-it-yourself means of getting the needed minerals into your body.

So study the cell salts for yourself, referring to the articles and books that accompany this chapter. You will find the information short, concise and intriguing, and I hope as rewarding for you as it has been for others.

HOW LONG DOES IT TAKE FOR CELL SALTS TO WORK?

Time for recovery resulting from the use of cell salts may vary from six weeks to three months, though Esther Chapman says: "But one does not need to wait for a full recovery to enjoy a measure of relief and greater ease."[4]

One person wrote: "Because I had never heard of the twelve cell salts, I was curious enough to order some, although I was skeptical, too. At first I didn't notice much change, but after using the all-in-one product, according to the label, for three months, I felt sure I was assimilating my vitamins and food a lot better because my hair and fingernails improved more than they had in all the years I have taken vitamins."[5]

INORGANIC VERSUS ORGANIC MINERALS

Is it true that many minerals, including those in the cell salts, are inorganic?

Yes, but analyses show that blood is composed of both inorganic and organic matter which, if it is supplied to the body regularly, is constantly being built into the body. Although the body is composed of both organic and inorganic elements, and the organic predominates, the organic cannot perform their proper function without the inorganic. Dr. William A. Albrecht, the late Professor Emeritus of Soils, College of Agriculture, University of Missouri, the dean of a life-time of research of trace minerals in soil and their effect on plants, animals and people, stated that though some minerals are insoluble (inorganic), *they become soluble on coming in contact with the mucous membranes of the body*. He also stated that the positively charged nutrients such as calcium, magnesium and potassium which may be insoluble to percolating water, are yet available to plant roots, due to cation or exchange. Thus he says the insoluble can become available through the exchange transformation to water; consequently *the insoluble becomes available nourishment*. He added that natural plant growth emphasizes the fact that the inorganic (considered insoluble) as well as the highly organic (soluble) are both *biochemically active*. Dr. Albrecht added that chelation (discussed later) may explain why nature can transform an insoluble element into a biochemically active one.

Any biochemistry textbook will tell you the same thing: both organic and inorganic elements occur in the body and both are needed to rebuild the constant wear and tear and degeneration of the body. Phosphorus, for instance, is not only present in inorganic combinations (such as bones, teeth and blood) but in many organic combinations. Inorganic and organic elements are in equilibrium with each other and come from the food we eat and the beverages we drink. In addition, my textbook adds: "Many enzymes require small quantities of inorganic elements for their activity."[6]

BEWARE OF TOXIC METALS

There are a few minerals, known as heavy metals, that are causing trouble for us because they are polluting our atmosphere and are highly toxic.

For example, we hear on all sides about lead poisoning (which has been found to cause brain damage, among other ailments), mercury poisoning, and, more recently, cadmium poisoning. We have held our breath and hoped they would go away. They haven't. They now exist in the polluted air, the water, the soil and the food grown in it. Dr. Harvey Ashmead, Ph.G., Ph.D., and a veterinarian, recently took a trip by car from Salt Lake City to Chicago. He stopped at invervals to take samples of soil. He even took samples of snow in the high Rockies where there was little or no civilization. There were 1,000 samples in all. He found evidence of lead pollution in all 1,000 samples.

Although many insist this lead is harmless inorganic lead, Dr. Ashmead does not agree. He says it is emitted into our atmosphere and deposited on snow, trees, brush, grass and soil and finally finds its way through plants into animals and people, or is inhaled directly from the air.

Other heavy toxic metals are mercury and cadmium. One symptom of such metal poisoning is an eczema between the fingers, with itching, small blisters, peeling and eventually rawness of the skin.

LEAD

The heavy metal lead has been found in waters contaminated by industrial waste; in turn, the fish from these waters have been found to be contaminated. Lead accumulates in the atmosphere from auto fuels; it is carried great distances by winds and is deposited in soils. Insecticides, phosphate fertilizers and wastes from various smelting operations also contaminate soils with lead, which in turn contaminates the food grown in that soil. However, according to a study done in Washington, D.C., the lead in contaminated food is retained in the blood to a far lesser extent than is atmospheric lead. As a result of breathing atmospheric lead, the auto fumes on the street, "Washington, D.C., is now considered the lead poisoning Capital, thanks to Detroit."[7] Lead-free gas is a partial solution: lead in the topsoil of Los Angeles has been found to be 3,000 parts per million, whereas in Moscow, where leaded gas is not used, the soil contains only 19 parts per million.

In addition to eczema, mentioned above, symptoms of lead poisoning include abdominal distress, diarrhea, general aches and pains, nausea and vomiting, constipation, neurological symptoms, paralysis, convulsions, headaches, depression and irritability. The cause of these disturbances is often overlooked by doctors.

Dr. Ashmead reports the case of a forty-five-year-old woman who had been suffering from depression, muscular aching, fatigue, nausea, vomiting and shooting pains in her head. She had suffered discomfort for a long time. Because the symptoms were typical of many other conditions, no doctor seemed able to diagnose the cause of her trouble. Finally a sample of her hair was sent to a laboratory that tests hair for mineral content (through doctors, only). An alarming amount of lead was found in the hair sample. The cause was traced to the woman's habit of drinking coffee from a pewter (silver-lead) cup. (Other forms of lead poisoning have been traced to unglazed pottery colored with a pigment containing lead.)

The treatment used by the woman's doctor eliminated the lead from her body.

FLUORIDES

Fluorides in the form of sodium fluoride pollute both air and water. They pollute the air through industrial smoke-stack emission. As we learned earlier, fluoride is an industrial by-product that can pollute water. The effects of this substance, identified as a poison, have been found to be cumulative. The Natural Food Associates of Atlanta, Texas, warn: "If your water supply is fluoridated, do not eat foods cooked in it or drink beverages made with it."[8] Symptoms of fluoride poison, according to Jonathan Forman, M.D., include the following:[9]

Sharp stomach pains
Nausea and bowel irritability and spasticity
Arthritic pains in lower spine, back stiffness
Migraine-like headaches
Loss of muscular power plus numbness in arms and legs
Mouth ulcers (worse if using fluoridated toothpaste)
Dryness of mouth and excessive thirst
Vision disturbances
Kidney damage and bladder stones
Occasionally, mental disturbances, loss of memory and inability to concentrate
Extreme fatigue
Allergic skin reactions

MERCURY

Mercury has been found in the air and the soil, as well as in water. Dr. Henry A. Schroeder wrote: "The earth's surface, both crust and sea water, has always contained mercury. Mercury is in river water that flows into the sea; the concentration is small: 6.68 to .8 parts per billion parts of water. Mercury precipitates in sea water, sinking to the ocean floor, leaving only .01 to .03 parts per million remaining in the sea water itself."[10]

Dr. Schroeder said that mercury is a constituent of every living thing. Life began in the sea, which has always contained mercury. Because oceans are neither polluted nor contaminated by mercury, ocean fish are not polluted, regardless of the mercury in their flesh. Thus ocean fish, tuna, swordfish, flounder, cod, haddock and halibut are safe to eat, he insists.

Dr. Schroeder added that *methyl mercury* (an industrial unnatural product) is entirely different, that it is highly toxic. If it is dumped in relatively confined waters (lakes and rivers) it can enter the food chain and people eating a lot of fish can be poisoned. Dr. Schroeder also warned against methyl and ethyl mercury treated seeds.

Tuna caught sixty-two to ninety-three years ago (preserved in cans) was tested by University of California chemists and found to contain as much mercury as found in today's ocean catch. Even a swordfish caught twenty-five years ago contained about the same amount of mercury as a swordfish caught today. The consensus is that ocean fish are little affected by mercury, and what mercury is present is in natural form. Scientists at the University of Wisconsin found that, even if tuna does contain mercury, this metal is deactivated by another metal—selenium.

A less favorable finding came from a study of South-west England and South Wales. It showed that 80 percent of the mercury found *was* methyl mercury, the highly toxic type. Shellfish contained the most; tuna the least.[11]

An explanation has been suggested by Swedish scientists, who discovered that certain bacteria are able to convert metallic mercury into organic compounds. These scientists suggest that algae absorbed the bacteria, fish ate the algae, and man ate the fish.[12] Through this food chain, mercury concentration was increased as much as 10,000 times. However, Dr. Schroeder did not agree that these findings denote a dangerous contamination of ocean fish.

Symptoms of methyl mercury poisoning include the following:

Damage to the nervous system
Mental disturbance
Loss of balance, and impaired walking
Disturbances in speech, sight and hearing
Difficulty in swallowing
Certain types of brain degeneration

According to Dr. Schroeder, the longer a person lives, the less mercury he stores in his body.

He stated: "The body can lose much methyl mercury in three months and almost all of it in ten years, except for brain damage. Brain damage is irreparable."[13]

CADMIUM

Cadmium is a real troublemaker. It is found mainly in water and soil and thus in foods. Cadmium is also present in the air coming from coal dust and smoke, petroleum and some gasolines. There is also a lot of cadmium in tin and aluminum cans. Probably, according to Dr. Schroeder, the source most common to many people is corroded galvanized pipes. He said soft water will corrode these pipes and hard water won't. He believed, therefore, that we should make our soft water harder by adding magnesium and calcium salts.

Watch out for cadmium pigments in cadmium red or yellow on poorly glazed pottery. As for foods, cadmium is not absorbed well if there is plenty of zinc present. Zinc occurs in the germ and the bran of grain, whereas cadmium is distributed throughout the grain. This is why *wholegrain* products are a safeguard against cadmium poisoning. Sugar as well as other processed foods such as instant coffee and instant tea contain cadmium, Dr. Schroeder said.[14] It also enters the body via cigarette smoke.

Cadmium as an air pollutant can cause emphysema, chronic bronchitis and lung fibrosis. The main result of too much cadmium is high blood pressure, which may lead to heart attacks and strokes.

COPPER

A dietary excess of copper is now found to be common in the United States. This is confirmed by the finding of copper in high amounts in some hair analysis.

There is a scarcity of tests on the effects of excess copper. Yet, as one journal states: "There is considerable more risk of copper toxicity than of copper deficit in man."[15] One finding is that copper is distributed through the teeth and may soften the enamel.[16]

Dr. Carl Pfeiffer, an expert in neuropsychiatry, states that there is increasing evidence that the majority of schizophrenic cases is caused by a lack of zinc and too much copper in the body. He explains that most people have too much copper in their bodies as a result of drinking water from copper pipes, eating foods cooked in copper utensils (the contact with copper pans also instantly destroys the vitamin C in foods), or perhaps by taking copper in vitamin supplements. He adds that 80 percent of the patients suffering from schizophrenia who were studied, were found to have a deficiency of zinc and an excess of copper and iron in their body tissues.

How can we protect ourselves? Dr. Henry Schroeder supplied one answer; Dr. Albrecht supplies another. Processed foods, said Dr. Schroeder, contain few minerals. When the food is rich in the major and trace minerals, the heavy metals are better resisted. To prevent the invasion of the heavy toxic metals, the food and the body should be filled to capacity with all minerals. Dr. Schroeder said that the milling of wheat into refined flour removes 40 percent of the chromium, 86 percent of the cobalt, 68 percent of the copper, 78 percent of the zinc and 48 percent of the molybdenum. Refined carbohydrates (white flour, white rice and white sugar) have had most of the minerals removed, but whole foods, including whole grains and brown rice, are more likely to contain the minerals in adequate amounts.

Dr. Albrecht, on the other hand, states that these (processed) foods cannot and do not contain their full quota of minerals *if the soil is deficient,* as it usually is. Thus our need for organically raised foods is imperative in this new era of pollution. Minerals in the proper proportion can assure us of sound bones and muscles, strong teeth, steady nerves, a keen mind, firm skin and healthy glands and organs.

Some doctors (including Dr. Pfeiffer) are using the chelated minerals to establish mineral balance, thus eliminating the excesses of copper, lead or iron, and at the same time providing zinc, manganese and other minerals that are in short supply.

It is important to repeat that, according to Dr. Schroeder, foods rich in balanced trace minerals will help the body resist the accumulation of the unwanted metals, and thus prevent resulting illness. But this food must be raised on rich mineralized soil. Soil depleted of minerals is empty soil, producing empty food in which the unwanted metals can accumulate.

ANTIDOTES FOR HEAVY METALS

Detection of heavy metals in the body can be accomplished by hair testing.

There are a few antidotes for the toxic, heavy metals:

For lead poisoning: Vitamin C (ascorbic acid). One study showed that five men who were given ascorbic acid eliminated lead acetate in their urine.[17]

Dr. Carlton Fredericks suggests large amounts of calcium daily. (The amount found in one quart of milk or four ounces of cheese, tahini or sesame butter, which are available at health stores.)[18]

Homeopathic remedies containing platinum, alum and petroleum. When ordering, state why you wish these substances, and the correct potency will be given you by the homeopathic pharmacy.

For cadmium poisoning: Vitamin C (ascorbic acid). In an FDA study, birds developed anemia after exposure to cadmium. Large doses of vitamin C reversed it.[19]

Camphora, a homeopathic remedy, is another possibility.

Zinc acetate. One study showed that pregnant mice exposed to cadmium were protected by injections of zinc acetate.[20]

For mercury poisoning: Hepar Sulph, 6x potency, a homeopathic remedy.

For copper poisoning: Hepar Sulph., 6x potency, a homeopathic substance.

For aluminum poisoning: Ipecac, 6x potency, a homeopathic
substance. Aluminum poisoning has been found more
widespread than is usually suspected.

THE NEWER CHELATED MINERALS

Perhaps the best overall protection against the heavy,
toxic metals are the chelated minerals.

Both Dr. M. L. Scott of Cornell University and Dr.
Harvey Ashmead have found that chelated minerals are
three times better assimilated than ordinary inorganic
minerals. Tests with hens given chelated minerals have
showed that the hens laid more eggs. Experiments with
200,000 horses, cows, pigs and sheep showed that these
new chelated minerals produce better mineral balance
and better growth of young animals. In some cases they
reduced disease. The late John J. Miller, Ph.D., has done
pioneer work with the chelates, especially on humans.[21]

What is chelation? The late William Seroy explained:
"The process of chelation is the means of surrounding or
enclosing a mineral atom by a larger protein molecule.
This process changes the positive ionic (electrolyte) charge
to a negative ionic charge, making it more acceptable
through the villi of the intestines into the bloodstream.
Thus it is transported to the cells which need and use
these minerals more easily and efficiently."

Dr. Ashmead states guardedly: "Preliminary research
indicates that organic chelated metals may have value in
altering heavy metal metabolism within the animal. Con-

siderable research needs to be accomplished in this area before a definite conclusion can be made."[22] Dr. Ashmead believes that theoretically any trace mineral can displace other metals according to their valence.

As one example, Dr. Ashmead was called upon, in the capacity of veterinarian as well as mineral expert, to diagnose a herd of sick sheep. He found that they had wandered into a pasture where the inorganic zinc content was too high, accounting for their illness. He gave them chelated iron, which displaced the excess iron, and the sheep recovered within two or three days.

This type of imbalance can occur in people, too. Dr. Pfeiffer, of the Brain Bio Center in Princeton, New Jersey, reports that of 300 schizophrenic patients who had been confined in mental institutions, more than 95 percent improved and returned home after trace element therapy. Dr. Pfeiffer believes that schizophrenia is primarily a biochemical disorder in the brain and that trace elements play a key role in maintaining a sound mind.

Fortunately, he says, the treatment is simple in effect: chelated iron will replace inorganic zinc, zinc will replace copper. Manganese helps, too. Dietary supplements of zinc and manganese can apparently eliminate the deficiency of these metals and can apparently displace copper in the body.

Although the chelated minerals include to date only calcium, phosphorus, magnesium, potassium, manganese, zinc, copper, iodine and cobalt, they are of tremendous help in protecting against the toxicity of the heavy metals. Vitamin E can be taken simultaneously with the iron in chelated minerals. Chelated minerals are gradually reaching the offices of nutritionally oriented doctors and health stores. Several laboratories now analyze samples of human hair in order to determine a deficiency or excess of minerals in the body. These deficiencies or excesses are usually corrected with the chelated minerals.

The value of this laboratory work is illustrated by this example: the laboratory found a critical shortage of certain minerals in a patient. Realizing that some time had already elapsed since the hair sample was taken and mailed to them by the doctor, and that more time would elapse before the analysis could reach the doctor, again by mail, the laboratory phoned the doctor. They advised giving the missing minerals *immediately*, since the laboratory considered the mineral at absolute zero level, thus a matter of life and death. The doctor answered, "The patient died this morning!"

Not all people are as low in minerals as this patient, but it does show how important it is for the average person to keep up the intake of minerals constantly.

A NEW APPROACH

There is a breakthrough in information about minerals. Nutritionists, following the results of available research, have always warned that minerals taken into the body must be both complete and in perfect balance. It now turns out that this concept is not necessarily true. Just as the early alchemists attempted to turn the baser metals into gold, it appears now, with proof, that the body can take certain minerals already present and transform them into other minerals. The source of this information, which has upset previous teaching, is a book called *Biological Transmutations*, by Louis Kervran, an active member of the New York Academy of Sciences, and a French researcher in chemistry and biochemistry.[23] Some accept the theory; others don't.

However this book has caused quite a stir, upsetting the applecart of previous beliefs in mineral nutrition. It can be of great interest to the average man; it is *must* reading for doctors and nutritionists. The book contains startling findings. If you need iron, take organic manganese, which will make the iron for you. If you need calcium, take organic silica. Through the addition of silica, the book states, "spectacular results have been obtained in the repairing of broken bones."

The book is replete with examples of this transmutation process. In one case, chickens, which could not get limestone for calcium, pecked at mica (a form of silica) in the soil and produced strong calcium-rich eggshells without calcium. And sea life, put in sea water from which all limestone had been removed, grew calcium-rich shells without calcium. Silica, incidentally, is found in the herb horsetail. Silica is also one of the cell salts known as Silicea.

The ability of the body to transmute minerals does not mean we should be careless about our intake of minerals. We *do* need them all. But neither should we panic when we cannot at times get all the minerals, nor should we worry about imbalances. If any are missing, the body will temporarily take over and manufacture what it needs from the others present. To take advantage of a hair analysis, be sure the laboratory which does it is reliable, with many years of successful experience behind it.

This brings us to the universal source of minerals since the world began: water.

SAFE DRINKING WATER

We have always known that a man can live for an

extended time without food, but not without water. Did you ever stop to reason why? It is because water contains minerals, a source of nourishment for the body. The more minerals in the water, the harder the water; the fewer the minerals, the softer the water.

Dr. Schroeder, already mentioned as internationally renowned for his mineral and trace element research, has established a finding, which has been confirmed by others throughout the world: that hard water rich in minerals, is found to cause less heart disease than soft water with few minerals. (Distilled water or artificially softened water has had practically all minerals removed.) Scientists also agree that when mineral-free water is taken, it leaches out of the body what minerals already exist there. This is apparently due to an ion exchange within the body, through the membranes.

If you have read that someone has died of heart disease because of drinking hard well water (a gold mine these days) remember that one case does not make a law any more than one swallow makes a summer. Don't blame the water. Hard water has been shown to be beneficial to millions. Blame, rather, the individual who drank the water. It might have been due to lack of assimilation. Hydrochloric acid is necessary for the proper assimilation of calcium and iron. If this acid is lacking, these minerals cannot be used and may be stored in unwanted places such as joints, causing arthritis, and in hearts.

One of the best examples of the effect of water on health is that of the Hunzas. The water where they live is so full of minerals, largely inorganic, that it is not only murky, but the sediment settles at the bottom of the glass when it is allowed to stand. Yet these people have been known for the best health of any people in the world.

Researchers consider their water greatly responsible. Heart disease is practically unknown. I have been told, however, that the Hunzas are ashamed of their water, and when some VIP's visit them, they serve them clear, mineral-free water in order to make a good impression on those from more "civilized" countries.

It is indeed true that today much of our water is polluted, either from heavy metals, insecticides or fluorides. In addition, too much chlorine and other types of contaminants make the water brackish, unpleasant to smell and taste. Unfortunately, many people in their desire for safe drinking water, are using distilled water. Yet *distilled water has no minerals at all;* and tests with humans have shown serious results from drinking it, because it leaches minerals from the body.[24]

Dr. Hazel Parcells, a Ph.D. nutritionist, says: "We found that using distilled water, as well as water from water softeners for drinking and cooking caused muscle weakness, the heart being one of the first victims of this poor mineral balance. Also the general muscle tone throughout the body was very poor. The blood chemistry of these people who drank such water showed a deficiency of calcium and other supportive minerals." This finding is in agreement with scientific tests around the world.

It is understandable that those who have unacceptable drinking water should wish to remove the contaminants. Distilling the water at home can accomplish this safely, provided that the minerals are restored to the lifeless distilled water. This can be done, but before I give you the formula, you need to know why this formula can be so effective: another type of water is needed to help out.

SEA WATER

Charles Ahlson reported the value of giving sea water to plants, animals and people. He said both bursitis and arthritis responded to drinking sea water.[25] George W. Crane, M.D., confirms this. He says: "It is entirely possible that water-soluble trace elements may prove the greatest medical innovation in preventing such ailments that have appeared in the twentieth century."

As we said earlier, your blood stream contains, by actual analysis, the identical minerals found in sea water. In cases of emergency, when blood for transfusions was unavailable, doctors have given transfusions of sea water. They found that the patient recovered on sea water as well as on blood transfusions.

Dr. Fritz Kahn tells us that if a human being were squeezed like a lemon, at least eleven gallons of water would be obtained with the same minerals and in the same proportion as ocean water.

Dr. Crane tells of the effect of sea water on his father-in-law, ninety-six years old, who had been bedfast and chairfast for ten years, with an arthritic hip. After taking sea water for four months, Grandpa got out of his invalid chair and began hobbling around; he also perked up mentally as well as physically. Dr. Crane said: "It seemed as if some miracle had happened. Maybe ocean water is the real 'fountain of youth' for it contains all the water-soluble elements on this earth." Dr. Crane is not only an M.D., but a Ph.D., and the author of the syndicated newspaper column, "The Worry Clinic." He names twenty-two common diseases that could be prevented by drinking sea water.

Most people do not drink sea water straight. They add a little to their regular drinking water. For those who insist on drinking distilled water, adding sea water to distilled water restores the missing minerals somewhat and does not interfere with the flavor. But beware of getting sea water yourself from the ocean's edge if near civilization; it can be contaminated. Safe sea water may be obtained thirty or more miles out at sea from the greatest depth possible. It can also be bought from health stores in filtered, unheated form. (Heating and other processing remove many of the minerals.)

Lee Hall, a Ph.D. in physiology, tells the true story of an elderly couple who outperformed all the younger people on Dr. Hall's staff in miles of hard tramping during ecology field trips. The man was seventy-five years old, his wife was sixty-five. Yet they outdistanced with ease the people in their forties and fifties. Not only did this couple have more energy, but they did not complain of the back and leg and joint problems that bothered many of the younger group. Finally, Dr. Hall asked the two for their "secret." They gave it gladly. They told him they had taken a tablespoon of sea water on their cereal every morning for forty years.

If you are a coffee drinker, you might follow the lead of coffee connoisseurs who believe that salt enhances the flavor. By adding a teaspoon of sea water to your morning cup of coffee you can gain both flavor and minerals. In the same general way, you can convert your distilled water, if you use it, to mineralized water, which will NOT leach the minerals from your body. Here is the formula, which I have had tested in the laboratory:

To a half gallon of distilled water, add four teaspoons of commercially filtered, bottled sea water (available at health food stores), or, to one pint of distilled water, add one eighth teaspoon of whole, ground sea salt. As mentioned before, this whole sea salt, which includes all minerals, comes from France or Belgium and is found in health food stores.

I wish all distilling companies would share this formula with their customers. The flavor is palatable and improves upon refrigeration. And the needed minerals are present.

We dare not take the chance of depending on foods as our only source of minerals. We should fortify ourselves with a rich supply of natural minerals from the sources I have named: whole sea salt, kelp, sea water, cell salts, alfalfa and chelated minerals.

Not only will a rich supply of minerals taken from these sources (perhaps in combination to ensure all needed factors) protect you against pollution by the toxic metals and other dangerous contaminants.[26] The minerals will also "charge your batteries" for better health.

REFERENCES

1. Charles B. Ahlson. *Health from the Sea and Soil.* Jericho, N.Y.: Exposition Press, 1962.

2. *Health Saver.* Spring, 1958, p. 17.

3. J. B. Chapman. *Dr. Schuessler's Biochemistry.* London, England: New Era Laboratories, Ltd., 1961.

4. Esther Chapman. *How to Use the Twelve Tissue Salts.* Paperback edition. New York: Pyramid Publications, 1971.

5. *Organic Consumer Report.* June 13, 1972.

6. Benjamin Harrow and Abraham Mazur. *Textbook of Biochemistry.* Seventh edition. Philadelphia: W. J. Saunders, 1958.

7. *Rodale's Health Bulletin.* March 4, 1972.

8. *Natural Food and Farming.* December, 1971.

9. *Ibid.*

10. Henry A. Schroeder. *Pollution, Profits and Progress.* Brattleboro, Vt.: Stephen Greene Press, 1971.

11. *Journal of the Association of Public Analysts.* Vol. 9, pp. 76–85. 1971.

12. Louise B. Young. *Power Over People.* Paperback edition. New York: Oxford University Press, 1974.

> *See also* Boyce Rensberger. "Mercury and Man; a Puzzle for Ecologists." *The New York Times,* News Analysis, p. 30. May 21, 1971.

13. Henry A. Schroeder, *op. cit.*

14. *Ibid.*

15. *American Journal of Clinical Nutrition,* October, 1972.

16. *American Journal of Pathology,* Vol. 50, p. 861. 1967.

17. *Science.* Vol. 173, pp. 820–827. 1971.

18. *The Carlton Fredericks Newsletter of Nutrition.* May 1, 1972.

19. *Prevention.* June, 1971.

20. *Reproductive Fertility.* Vol. 10, p. 263. 1965.

21. *Journal of Applied Nutrition.* Spring, 1972.

22. *Ibid.*

23. Louis Kervran. *Biological Transmutations.* Paperback edition. Binghamton, N.Y. 13902: Swan House Publishing, 1972.

24. Linda Clark. *Light On Your Health Problems.* Paperback edition. New Canaan, Conn.: Keats Publishing, 1972.

25. Charles B. Ahlson, *op. cit.*

26. Linda Clark. *Are You Radioactive?* Paperback edition. Old Greenwich, Conn.: Devin-Adair, 1973.

See also:

Len Mervyn. *Minerals & Your Health.* New Canaan, Conn.: Keats Publishing, 1981.

17
Cholesterol, Fats and Oils

Whenever I hear someone say smugly, "I am on a low cholesterol diet," I blow my top. The low cholesterol diet is a snare and delusion, and it went out of date years ago.

My bewildered listeners have asked, "But isn't cholesterol dangerous?" Of course it can be dangerous, but refusing to eat foods containing it is more dangerous. If you don't eat cholesterol, your body will still manufacture it. Cholesterol is necessary for the good performance of your sex glands, is involved in bile salts production and the natural assimilation of vitamin D formed on the skin by sunshine.

DOESN'T CHOLESTEROL FROM FOOD CAUSE THE BLOOD'S CHOLESTEROL TO RISE, LEADING TO HEART ATTACKS?

Not necessarily. Cholesterol has been found to go up during stress periods or worry (accountants are shown to have a higher cholesterol during income tax preparation time). Exercise can lower cholesterol. Excessive sugar and smoking have been found to raise it. J. D. Ratcliffe states: "Many physicians are today questioning the importance of cholesterol as a leading factor in the heart disease problem. Although high blood levels of cholesterol are usually found in people with heart trouble, there is a growing suspicion that this may be not cause and effect, but purely associative. Says one researcher: 'We could as well note that countries which have the most telephones and flush toilets also have the most heart disease.' "[1]

Dr. John Miller believed there may be more danger of the increased manufacture of cholesterol as a result of its being avoided in the diet, than if people ate it, because the body has to work so hard to compensate, by making more cholesterol.

One of the biggest scares and biggest myths is that you shouldn't eat eggs for fear they will raise your cholesterol. Studies have shown that eating as many as twelve eggs a day has not increased the cholesterol level. As a matter of fact, eggs have a built-in cholesterol dissolver, called lecithin, which we will discuss later.

Isn't cholesterol dangerous when it rises in the blood? Can it plug up the arteries and thus lead to a coronary attack? The answer to both questions can be yes, but the way to prevent this rise is not to avoid foods that contain cholesterol. There are better and easier ways to prevent the rise of cholesterol in your body and avoid cholesterol deposits. Cholesterol is a waxy yellowish substance present in every cell of the body. It is especially rich in the spinal cord, nerves and brain—it makes up to 10 percent of the brain's weight. Even when it is completely eliminated from the diet, it still continues to circulate in the blood after it has been manufactured within your body, mostly by the liver. It is only when it accumulates in the arteries that concern is warranted. But this concern often leads to a still more ridiculous diet: a non-fat diet.

Cholesterol is usually associated with fats, which may supply some of the raw material from which cholesterol is made. For this reason, or because many people believe that eating fat makes them fat, they go on a non-fat diet. Wrong again. This is really hazardous. Why? Let me explain.

To begin with, one study showed that a fat-free diet given to rats caused scaly feet, dandruff, sores and bleeding of the skin. Another study showed that a fat-free diet for rats produced more, rather than less, cholesterol deposits in their arteries.[2] A nine-year study found that people who ate no fat at all had the highest blood fat levels, whereas those who ate 70 percent fat in their diet had the lowest.[3] As mentioned, Bucknell University found that a fat-free diet can cause gallstones.[4] Fat is needed to make the gallbladder work. With little or no fat, it does not empty. Finally, as you have already learned, the fat-soluble vitamins (A, D, E and K) cannot function in the body without fats.

Dr. Arthur M. Master, quoted in the *Journal of the American Medical Association*, says: "Many factors other than diet play a role in coronary disease, including emotion and behavior patterns, lack of physical exercise, excessive smoking, heredity and sex. Many non-fat nutrients appear to be involved. . . . In the present incomplete state of our knowledge, a drastic change in the diet is not justified."

Dr. Wilfrid E. Shute, the heart specialist, writes: "There is much evidence to suggest that there is no relationship between dietary fat and coronary artery disease. . . . Similarly, the commonly held relationship between atherosclerosis and coronary thrombosis has no validity."[5]

Arteriosclerosis vs. atherosclerosis: what is the difference? Arteriosclerosis, often called hardening of the arteries, is actually a thickening of the artery walls. Atherosclerosis is a clogging or filling up of the arteries, sometimes by fatty or cholesterol products. For suggested treatment, see chapter 18.

WHAT ABOUT THAT OLD IDEA THAT EATING FAT MAKES YOU FAT?

Richard Mackarness, M.D., of England says that starch and sugar (carbohydrates) are the real causes of obesity.[6] Plenty of fat people, he says, also have low blood cholesterols and many thin people have high cholesterols. One nutritional journal reports that there is more weight lost on a high fat diet than on a high carbohydrate diet.[7] The inability to utilize carbohydrates apparently converts carbohydrates to fat, whereas the fat we eat acts as a wick to burn fat away in the body. It also staves off hunger. The high fat diet has appeared under many names. One name, the Du Pont Diet, originated because the diet was tried at the Du Pont plant under the supervision of Alfred Pennington, M.D. The results were dramatic.

Twenty overweight men and women were allowed to eat all the meat and fat they wished. These dieters reported that they felt well, relished their meals and were never hungry between meals. Many of them were amazed at their increased energy; none complained of fatigue. These overweight men and women lost an average of twenty-two pounds each (some as much as fifty-four total pounds, some as little as nine pounds, according to their need to lose) within three and one-half months. Those who had high blood pressure at the beginning of the diet were told by their doctors that their blood pressure drop paralleled their drop in weight.

Actually this diet was the forerunner of the low-carbohydrates diet, permitting not more than 60 gm. of carbohydrates, but unlimited protein, salads, butter and many fruits (including berries, orange and grapefruit, fresh pears, plums and peaches). Oils, as in salad dressings, were encouraged.

Adelle Davis had been puzzled for years by people who were not only overweight, but whose ankles, legs and thighs were swollen with water retention even though their protein intake was high. She learned that when two tablespoons of salad oil were added to their daily diet, they lost pounds. She concluded that eating too little fat is probably a major cause of overweight.[8]

This brings us to oils.

WHICH ARE THE BEST OILS TO EAT?

Vegetable oils are among our most important foods. Contrary to belief, fats as well as oils are not wholly unsaturated or saturated; they are both. (See the following table.) Polyunsaturated oils are more unsaturated than others (poly means more).

When unsaturated fatty acids predominate in a fat, the fat becomes liquid at room temperature. When saturated fats predominate they become solid at room temperature. Since the oils have greater solubilizing effect on fats, they tend to liquefy the fats in the human body, instead of being stored as deposits or plaques, which may clog the body's arteries. The oils highest in unsaturated fatty acids (the polyunsaturates) include safflower, corn, cod liver, sunflower, sesame and soybean oils.

FOOD FAT OR OIL		SATUR-ATED FATTY ACIDS	UNSAT-URATED FATTY ACIDS
MEATS:	Beef	48	44
	Lamb	56	40
	Rabbit	38	58
MILK FAT:	Cow	55	39
	Goat	62	33
	Human	46	44
POULTRY	Chicken (not skin)	32	64
AND EGGS:	Turkey (not skin)	29	67
	Chicken eggs	32	64
FISH:	Herring	19	77
	Salmon	15	79
	Tuna (fresh, or not packed in oil)	25	70
SEPARATED	Butter	55	33
FATS AND OILS:	Partly hardened margarine	26	57
	Cod liver oil	15	81
	Corn oil	10	84
	Cottonseed oil	25	71
	Soybean oil	15	80
	Sunflower oil	12	83
	Peanut oil	18	76
	Sesame oil	14	80
	Safflower oil	8	87
CEREALS	Whole wheat	14	76
AND GRAINS:	Millet	31	61
	Wheat germ	17	77
	Oats	22	74

SEEDS, VEGETABLES AND FRUITS:	Avocado pulp	20	69
	Chocolate	56	39
	Olives	11	84
	Pumpkin seed	17	78
	Sesame seed	14	80
	Soybeans	20	75
NUTS:	Almonds	8	87
	Brazils	20	76
	Cashews	17	78
	Coconut	86	8
	Filbert (hazelnut)	5	91
	Peanuts	28	72
	Walnuts	7	89
	Pecans	7	84

Chart courtesy of Edna Gwillim, B.S., nutrition consultant.

Oils can be "hardened" through hydrogenation, a process of converting a liquid fat into a solid fat by adding hydrogen atoms. They do not become liquid at room temperature. Unsaturated fats are liquid at far below the body temperature (98.6) or approximately at 60 degrees. Hydrogenated or solid fats melt only at 114 degrees or higher. Thus only those fats with a low melting point are easily utilized by the human body. Therefore, it is logical that these unsaturated oils are preferable to the hard fats, such as lard and similar shortenings.

But there is another criterion you should watch for.

IF YOU USE OIL, HOW IS THAT OIL PREPARED?

I used to believe, and had even written, that when an oil was labeled as being cold-pressed, it meant cold-pressed. I learned later that this is not necessarily so. There are three conventional methods of extracting oils from nuts, grains, beans, seeds or olives:

The hydraulic press method.

The expeller press method.

Solvent extraction.

Those oils made by the hydraulic press method are more likely to be cold-pressed. Sesame and olive oil are examples. The expeller press uses a large screw-type apparatus. The source material it presses to extract the oil has been heated twice: first by cooking to soften it before pressing, and again by the expeller itself, which generates tremendous heat when it exerts its pressure. Thus the expeller pressed oils are not truly cold-pressed.

The third method of extracting oils, solvent extraction, uses a chemical solvent to precipitate the oil. This solvent is a petroleum product, which may be similar to that used in gasoline: pentane, heptane, hexane, octane or trichloroethylene. Thus these oils are dissolved oils, not pressed oils, and the solvent, which leaves a dry residue, may remain in the oil. According to experts on the subject, these oils should not be allowed to enter the human body.[9]

But this is not the end of the indignities to which oil can be subjected. In order to make an oil "look pretty" or to make the flavor more bland, much oil is further refined. Most of this type of oil appears in supermarkets. To prepare it, after the extraction by one of the three processes mentioned above, it is heated. It is then sprayed with lye to neutralize the free fatty acids. After it is washed, it is heated again, then bleached and reheated. (More and more valuable nutrients have now gone down the drain.) Strangely enough, this refined oil becomes rancid more easily than less refined oil because of the removal of the stabilizing factors.

Hydrogenation is a final insult to oils. According to *Prevention:* "Hydrogenation is a chemical process that many fats are subjected to, to solidify them. It is very destructive of valuable food elements. Margarine is a hydrogenated fat. Lard and other solid shortenings have been added to some peanut butter to improve its consistency (to prevent the oil from separating from it). Practically anything you buy in the way of processed foods like crackers, bakery products, pies and pastries have been made with hydrogenated fats."[10]

What oils are the safest? Except for sesame and olive oils (the best, first-pressed olive oil is usually labeled as "virgin"), there are only the crude oils, which have had little or no processing. However, the crude oils are often too strong in flavor to be palatable.

WHAT IS THE DIFFERENCE BETWEEN COLD-PRESSED AND COLD-PROCESSED OIL?

The terms "cold-pressed oils" and "expeller oils" are synonymous in the vegetable oil industry. Cold-pressed only means that no external heat has been applied at the expeller. (It implies that no heat is applied before pressing, which is not necessarily the case.)

COLD-PROCESSED OIL

The term "cold-processed oils" means that no heat is applied or allowed to be generated before or during the process of extraction. That is, the oil is not heated at any step used in the extraction plant.

However, if the expeller used to extract the oil develops high enough pressure, part of the mechanical energy is changed into heat energy and the oil is heated. When this happens the term "cold-processed" is inaccurate and misleading.

In order to avoid this interchange of energy, the extraction of the oil under high pressure should be slow enough to allow the heat to dissipate naturally. Or some other means could be used to remove heat as it is generated, such as running cold water through the screw of the press. The oil thus remains unheated and can truly be called cold-processed.

The public is generally unaware of the type of oil it is using.

DOES HEATING UNSATURATED FATS TURN THEM INTO SATURATES?

No!

Frank B. Lachle, an authority on oil extraction, stated emphatically that there is a misconception being circulated about oils: that heating unsaturated oils resaturates them.[11] This is NOT true, he said. The molecule is changed by the heat, but saturation does not occur. It is true that heating oils to the smoking point can cause oxidation (rancidity), which has often been mentioned in the same breath as carcinogens (cancer-causers).

Now what about margarines? Should they be used? Are they better or worse than butter? Most margarines, in order to be firm at room temperature, contain hydrogenated oil, which is not as desirable as naturally liquid oil. Despite the advertising to the contrary, experts say that they will not lower your cholesterol. So if you use margarine, you might as well choose it mainly on the basis of taste. The better margarines are those that contain liquid oils (in addition to hydrogenated). They must be kept under refrigeration, both at the store and at home. Margarines that contain no fillers or preservatives, with the exception of lecithin, are preferable. It is possible to make both margarines and shortening that are 90 percent unhydrogenated.

IS IT SAFE TO EAT ANIMAL OR SATURATED FATS?

How can you eat fats safely? Which ones are acceptable? First, it is probably wise to trim off the visible fats from your meat. Even when these have been removed, meat (due to marbling) still contains 50 percent fat. There is a new trend in some of the supermarkets to stock and label meat as "fat," "medium" and "lean." It is about time, because farmers have too long been fattening their stock to increase pounds and therefore the cash return. When you cook meats, see that the fats drip off without smoking and can be discarded. Avoid deep fat fried foods that have been cooked in oils heated and reheated many times. Beware of synthetic or imitation ice cream. It is often only flavored shortening. If you cannot get natural ice cream made with raw certified milk, make your own.

WHAT OTHER PRECAUTIONS SHOULD
BE TAKEN?

When using oil, remember that once a bottle of oil (buy the least refined, usually at health stores only) is opened, it should be kept refrigerated so that it will not become rancid. *The more oil you use, the more vitamins E and*

C you need, to prevent the oil's oxidation (rancidity) in the body.

And don't avoid butter. Most experts now agree that because butter is a natural product, and is completely liquid at body temperature, it should not be shunned. The fat experts I know use butter almost exclusively, with oils for cooking and for salads. Peanut butter, if it is made of peanuts and salt only, is fine. It is a good way to use a fat as a between meal snack to avoid hunger as well as to prevent weight gain. Take it straight or stuff a stalk of celery with it.

If you really wish to lower your cholesterol and prevent cholesterol plugs in your arteries, instead of going on a cholesterol-free or fat-free diet, which you know is not the answer, take lecithin! In Chapter 13, you learned that choline dissolves cholesterol. Lecithin contains choline in abundant amounts and is an excellent cholesterol emulsifier or dissolver, as well as a safe one. Lecithin is available in three forms: liquid, powder and granules as described in the next chapter. Just to show you one example of lecithin's value (among thousands of cases): one nutritionist conducted a study of patients with high cholesterol in which meat fat was not cut off, one or two eggs per day were eaten, plus butter and whole milk with heavy cream. Vegetable oil was used on salads and brewer's yeast was added to provide choline. One to three tablespoons of lecithin were taken daily. In every case, the cholesterol dropped to normal.

REFERENCES

1. J. D. Ratcliffe. "Cholesterol: Guilty or Not Guilty." *Reader's Digest*. November, 1964.

2. Linda Clark. *Stay Young Longer.* Paperback edition. New York: Pyramid Communications, 1968.

3. *Ibid.*

4. *Ibid.*

5. Wilfrid E. Shute and Harald J. Taub. *Vitamin E for Ailing and Healthy Hearts.* Paperback edition. New York: Jove Books (BJ Publishing Group), 1972.

6. Richard Mackarness. *Eat Fat and Grow Slim.* New York: Doubleday, 1958; or Pocket Books, 1962.

7. *Nutrition Reviews.* October, 1962, p. 294.

8. Adelle Davis. *Let's Eat Right to Keep Fit.* Paperback edition. New York: New American Library, 1970.

9. Paul Hawken and Fred Rohe. "The Oil Story." Distributed by Organic Merchants c/o Erewhon Trading Co., 8003 Beverly Blvd., Los Angeles, Calif. 90048.

10. *Prevention.* November, 1958, p. 133.

11. Frank B. Lachle. "Are You Eating the Right Fats?" *National Health Federation Bulletin.* September, 1968.

See also:

Philip Goldberg. "The Great Cholesterol Controversy." *Executive Health,* 1978.

Carl C. Pfeiffer. "Cholesterol and the Frequently Maligned Egg." *Health Quarterly,* vol. 1, no. 1.

18
High-Power Foods

There are a few special foods that have long been called 'wonder foods" or "miracle foods." This is not quite the correct terminology, for it gives the impression that these foods are panaceas. These foods are merely richer in many more nutrients than most foods. While they will not cure everything, they can be likened to high octane gasoline versus regular: they deliver more pep and promote a greater output of energy. These foods have been pooh-poohed by some detractors, but as you will see by the analysis of some of them, there is proof that they are richer nutritionally, and can therefore deliver more power. By incorporating these foods into your diet, you can save eating many pounds, or large amounts of less potent foods that merely fill you up and perhaps add unwanted weight. They are also a good value, financially, because they are full of free vitamins, minerals and amino acids (protein factors), which would cost much more were you to buy them separately.

Let's consider them one by one.

LECITHIN

Lecithin, as we have previously discussed, helps to homogenize or emulsify cholesterol in the body. Lecithin is made of four factors: ordinary fat, unsaturated fatty acids, choline (the B vitamin) and phosphorus. It is pronounced *less-i-thin*. It is found in every cell of the body and should be kept there to help the body do its work effectively.

Because lecithin includes phosphorus, it is needed by the brain. It also is a natural tranquilizer because it is found in the myelin sheath that surrounds the nerves. And it is found in the heart, bone marrow, kidneys, liver and spinal cord. It is extremely necessary for the male sex glands because lecithin is lost with the sperm. Lecithin should be constantly replaced to prevent a deficiency in any of the important body functions.

Women will be delighted to learn that it helps to distribute body weight more evenly (taking it off where you don't want it and putting it where you do). It also helps to plump up the skin. Lecithin works slowly to accomplish its wonders, but it works exceedingly well. Cases of heart disturbance, high cholesterol, angina and myasthenia gravis have responded to lecithin. *Medical World News* has reported that it may be helpful in preventing gallstones.[1]

Roger J. Williams, Ph.D., confirms what we have been saying about the effect of lecithin on cholesterol. He says not to shun cholesterol foods but to "consume more lecithin." He cites the work of Lester M. Morrison, M.D., who found that the cholesterol levels in the blood of twelve patients were lowered when the patients consumed about an ounce of lecithin daily for three months.

Lecithin is made from soybeans. It is available in

three forms: liquid, powder and granules. The granules have been used for many years by Dr. Morrison and by Adelle Davis, who recommended three to six tablespoons daily to lower a high cholesterol level. She told of a ten-year-old girl with an abnormally high cholesterol level, as well as a heart condition. The girl was bedridden and had been given up by the doctors. Daily, several tablespoons of lecithin granules were sprinkled on her salads or added to juice, and she was given vitamins B and E and unsaturated oil. She recovered. Her cholesterol became normal and she was able to return to school.

Lecithin is tasteless in any form. Hans Wohlgemuth, a lecithin researcher, believes that liquid lecithin is effective in lesser amounts than the other forms. He believes that one teaspoonful taken morning and evening is enough to overcome a deficiency and keep it in the blood at all times for protection and prevention of lecithin-deficiency disturbances.[2]

Liquid lecithin is not easy to take until you get used to it. It looks like honey and pours like honey, but there the similarity ends. It certainly does not taste like honey. (It tastes like nothing.) It also tends to stick to the roof of the mouth. You can try it in, or followed by, a tart fruit juice. If you take it by the teaspoonful, it will stick to the spoon. I usually tip the can and estimate a teaspoonful as it flows into my mouth. Then I follow with a tart fruit juice or hot drink. (When you begin to follow the nutritional way of life, you cease to be fussy.) All types of lecithin are available at health stores.

PRODUCT INFORMATION OF LIQUID LECITHIN

(Analysis also applies generally to dry lecithin)
Each tablespoon (liquid) is the equivalent of approximately

1½ tablespoons of lecithin granules or one dozen 1200 mg. capsules of lecithin.

One tablespoon (15.5 grams) of liquid lecithin supplies approximately:

Calories	110
Protein	0 grams
Carbohydrate	1 gram
Fats and fatty acids	12 grams
Cholesterol	0 mg.
Sodium	5 mg.

Percentage of USRDA

Iron	6%
Vitamin E	6%
Phosphorus	25%
Magnesium	6%

Contains less than 2% of USRDA of vitamins A, C, thiamin, riboflavin, niacin, calcium.

Made of natural lecithin derived from unrefined soy bean oil, it has nothing removed, no added artificial colors, flavors or preservatives.

Courtesy of Midland Soya, Le Seuer, Minn. 56068

BREWER'S YEAST

Brewer's yeast is one of the biggest food finds of the century. This is not a calculated guess; it is a fact as proved with thousands upon thousands of cases of health improvement resulting from its use. A list of its contents explains why it is such a high-powered food. It contains all of the major B vitamins (except B-12, which can be especially bred into it), nineteen amino acids (making it a complete protein), and eighteen or more minerals. Except for vitamins A, E and C, which it lacks, it can be considered a whole food.

A more detailed list of its contents follows:

Vitamins B-1 or thiamin, B-2 or riboflavin, B-3 or niacin, B-6 or pyridoxine, choline, inositol, pantothenic acid, PABA and biotin. B-12 does not occur unless especially "bred" into nutritional yeast. Ask for it at health stores.

Protein (amino acids): lysine, tryptophane, histidine, phenylalanine, leucine, methionine, valine, glycine, alanine, aspartic acid, glutamic acid, proline, hydroxyproline, tryosine, cystine and arginine.

Minerals: calcium, phosphorus, potassium, magnesium, silicon, copper, manganese, zinc, aluminum, sodium, iron, tin, boron, gold, silver, nickel, cobalt and iodine.

Brewer's yeast, originally a by-product of beer, is a powdered, dried residue. It has been "killed" by heat; it will not cause bread to rise, or, by the same token, feed upon your intestinal vitamins and multiply in your body, creating gas. It may cause gas for some people, as any high protein food can, but the addition of hydrochloric acid (to be discussed in the next chapter) can prevent this problem. It is also true that like many other foods, it is an allergen for some people.

Brewer's yeast is becoming so popular as a food that it is now being made specifically for that purpose. It is often called nutritional yeast. Instead of being available in powder only, it is now made in large and small flake form. Both Adelle Davis and I have listed examples galore of the improvement of health through the use of brewer's yeast or nutritional yeast. I will mention here only one benefit, in addition to the value of being a good reducing food. It increases energy

I have tried yeast for energy myself and I have watched my children and grandchildren use it as a pick-up. My elder daughter, particularly, when she feels slightly fatigued, will automatically go to the yeast canister, kept beside the flour, and other natural food staples, stir a tablespoon or so into liquid and drink it down. Within about ten minutes a pickup is noted, which, unlike the temporary lift of coffee or tea, lasts for several hours. Most people begin with a teaspoon in fruit juice or tomato juice or hot bouillon, which blends with the slightly savory flavor of the yeast. Later, people work up gradually to one-fourth cup daily, and they no longer bother about putting it in juice, but add it to plain water and gulp it down.

Yeast flakes are somewhat milder in flavor, but it takes more of them to provide the equivalent of the powder. Yeast tablets are also available but it takes twenty-four tablets to equal one tablespoon of yeast powder or flakes. Health stores, of course, provide all forms. If you take separate B vitamins, which are almost always synthetic, it is very important to take brewer's yeast the same day. The yeast is a source of natural B vitamins, which prevents vitamin B imbalance.

Because brewer's yeast, like other protein foods, is high in phosphorus, it is advisable when taking it, to add extra calcium. (Phosphorus, a co-worker of calcium, can take the calcium out of the body with it, leaving a calcium deficiency.) The remedy for this is easy. Mix up your pound of yeast with one-fourth cup of calcium lactate powder (available at health or drug stores). Mix well and keep in any container. It need not be refrigerated. The calcium corrects the calcium-phosphorus imbalance so that leg or other cramps can be prevented. By having the mixture premixed, it is convenient when you want to use it quickly.

WHEAT GERM

Wheat germ is a superior food. The United States Department of Agriculture considers it an excellent food for the following reasons: "A grain of wheat, like all seeds, contains the nutriment needed for germination and growth of the seedling. Protein, minerals, B vitamins, fat and carbohydrates are present in the right proportion ... the germ or embryo contains a large proportion of the vitamins and protein of superior quality. White flour, as it is milled today ... has removed the germ, also the greater part of the minerals and vitamins and much of the protein."[3]

In a later yearbook it adds: "Losses in milling are even higher for some less familiar nutrients. For example, vitamin E is present in high concentrations in the oil of the wheat germ. Nearly all of this vitamin is removed with the germ."[4]

This tells the story of wheat germ in a nutshell. As we have said again and again: because the wheat germ is removed from bread and cereals to protect the shelf life, our bread and cereals are lacking vitamin E, which comes from wheat germ. Cattle, deprived of wheat germ and vitamin E, have dropped dead of heart disease. Many Americans are following suit. When the wheat-germ vitamin E was restored to the cattle feed, the deaths from heart disease ceased. This valuable nutrient is not restored to the food for people. They must take it on their own. Meanwhile, the Drs. Wilfrid E. and the late Evan V.

Shute have rehabilitated the hearts of thousands of people, with vitamin E.[5]

Wheat-germ oil has been tested by various laboratories on animals and humans, especially athletes. It has been found invaluable in building energy and outwitting fatigue. Both wheat-germ and wheat-germ oil, once opened, should be kept refrigerated to prevent rancidity. The raw wheat germ is less tasty but valuable for adding to baked products. The toasted type, usually vacuum-packed to prevent rancidity until opened, is more palatable and children love it when it is floated on top of milk as a cereal. It can also be used instead of bread crumbs for breading meat and vegetables, or added to meat loaf, breads, biscuits, muffins, waffles and hot cakes.

There is a newer type of wheat germ now available in most health stores. It is called a high potency embryo chunk-style wheat germ. This does not mean that it comes in chunks, but that it is not rolled flat. (The chunks are noticeable only under a magnifying glass.) This type is less subject to rancidity, due to underprocessing. Unfortunately, many people report an allergic reaction not only to wheat but to the wheat germ especially.

ANALYSIS OF WHEAT GERM

	(per ounce)
Vitamin B-1	.45 mg.
Vitamin B-2	.14 mg.
Vitamin B-3 (Niacin)	.5 mg.
Vitamin B-6	.45 mg.
Vitamin E	7.00 mg.
Oil	8.4%
Protein	23%

Copper	.4	mg.
Iron	2.5	mg.
Manganese	4.0	mg.

SUNFLOWER SEEDS

Most seeds are an excellent source of many nutrients, but sunflower seeds take the prize. Whenever your children, or you, feel the need for a snack to hold you together until mealtime, sunflower seeds are a natural. They are good for that four o'clock slump and save a low blood sugar reaction if taken with coffee. They are also said to be good for the eyes.

Sunflower seeds should be eaten hulled and raw. Cooking them causes a loss of some valuable nutrients. They should be refrigerated after opening. Otherwise they can become rancid. If a jar or other container of sunflower seeds should smell rancid, return it, explaining the reason to the health store operator. (He knows that rancid foods can be disturbing to health, even dangerous.)

If you are traveling and want something to nibble while you wait for a bus, train or plane, a few sunflower seeds will give you a lift within minutes. I always carry them with me. For victims of hypoglycemia (low blood sugar) they are invaluable. They raise the blood sugar naturally through the protein content and are much wiser to take than something sweet. Here is the analysis:

ANALYSIS OF SUNFLOWER SEEDS
PER 100 GRAMS OR ⅕ POUND

Phosphorus	860.0 mg.
Iron	6.0 mg.
Calcium	57.0 mg.
Iodine	0.07
Magnesium	347.0 mg.
Potassium	630.0 mg.
Manganese	25 ppm
Copper	20 ppm
Zinc	66.5
Sodium	.4
Vitamin A	68 I.U.
B Vitamins	
B-1 (Thiamin)	2.2 mg.
B-2 (Riboflavin)	0.28 mg.
B-3 (Niacin)	5.6 mg.
B-6 (Pyridoxine)	1.1 mg.
B-12	.04 mcg. per gm.
PABA	62. mg.
Biotin	0.067 mg.
Choline	216. mg.
Inositol	147. mg.
Folic acid	0.1 mg.
Pantothenic acid	2.2 mg.
Pantothenol	3.5 mg.
Vitamin D	92 USP units
Vitamin E	31 I.U.
Protein	25%
Sunflower oil	48.44%
(over 90% unsaturated)	

ALFALFA

Alfalfa is said to be one of the most complete and nutritionally rich of all foods tested. In addition to a fabulously high potency of vitamins as well as minerals, it is high in protein and contains every essential amino acid. Its antitoxin or detoxification properties surpass those of every food tested: liver, brewer's yeast and wheat germ. Although these foods, too, have antitoxin properties, alfalfa is superior in this respect. It has been found to provide resistance to disease and seems to help those ailments that end in "itis" such as arthritis. It also helps to prevent exhaustion and provides an excellent calcium-phosphorus ratio (2:1). A very few people seem to be allergic to alfalfa; watch it!

Alfalfa seems to be most effective when it has had the fiber removed before being pressed into tablets. (The fiber upsets some people's digestion.) Alfalfa is an outstanding natural product as the following analysis shows.

ANALYSIS OF DEHYDRATED ALFALFA

Vitamins		Per 100 Grams
A	up to	44,000 I.U.
D		1,040 I.U.
E		50 I.U.
K		15 I.U.
U		unknown
C		176 mg.
B-1		0.8 mg.
B-2		1.8 mg.
B-6		1.0 mg.
B-12		0.3 mcg.

Niacin	5 mg.
Pantothenic acid	3.3 mg.
Inositol	210 mg.
Biotin	033 mg.
Folic acid	0.8 mg.

Other Content

Fiber	25%
Protein	20%
Fat solubles	3%

Minerals

Phosphorus	250 mg.
Calcium	1,750 mg.
Potassium	2,000 mg.
Sodium	150 mg.
Chlorine	280 mg.
Sulfur	290 mg.
Magnesium	310 mg.
Copper	2 mg.
Manganese	5 mg.
Iron	35mg.
Cobalt	2.4 mg.
Boron	4.7 mg.
Molybdenum	2.6 ppm

Trace Minerals

Nickel
Strontium 90
Lead
Paladium

RICE POLISHINGS

Rice polish (or rice bran) is loaded with B vitamins. It is the outer covering removed from whole, brown, natural rice.

Rice polish has a mild flavor and its use is an excellent method of fortifying foods. Usually, after it is taken off the white rice, it is sold back to the public in vitamin preparations. It is less expensive, in the long run, to buy it in powder form at healthstores and add it to breads, biscuits, muffins, pie crust, meat loaf and cereals. It can be used cooked or uncooked. Cooking does not destroy its value. The best use of all is to cook and use the delicious whole brown rice.

CULTURED MILKS

The cultured milks are of great value for health. They help to stabilize the intestinal flora so that digestion is improved and many B vitamins can be synthesized in the intestines. After taking antibiotics, it is imperative to take acidophilus or one of the cultured milks, for the antibiotics kill the friendly intestinal flora that must be reestablished to encourage the return of health. In Italy, doctors routinely prescribe a cultured milk product when prescribing antibiotics.

The cultured milks include kefir, cultured buttermilk and yogurt. These can be purchased, but it is also possible to allow your own milk to clabber at room temperature; or with the aid of a starter which can be purchased from health stores, make your own. Kefir is liquid. Yogurt is more custard-like. Directions are supplied when you purchase the starter.[6]

There is some indication that, whereas powdered

skim milk has been used to make yogurt more solid, it is better to use a minimum because it is rich in galactose, an antagonist to vitamin B-2 (riboflavin). Animals made deficient in riboflavin have developed cataracts. Yogurt starter may be perverted by artificial additives (colorings and flavorings). Countries that have used it for generations for health use it plain.

Even so—many people are allergic to cow's milk in any form, due to a body lack of an enzyme called lactase, needed to neutralize lactose or milk sugar. This problem is now easily solved. Milk digestant tablets to be taken before using a milk product are available in health stores.

BLACKSTRAP MOLASSES

Blackstrap molasses is a food that you may hear belittled. Those who do not understand nutrition may consider blackstrap a fad. As we have said, no single food is a panacea; but blackstrap, as you will note in the accompanying analysis supplied to me by the medical profession, is a truly rich source of minerals and vitamins.

ANALYSIS

Five tablespoons of blackstrap molasses contain:

Calcium	258 mg.
Phosphorus	30 mg.
Iron	7.97 mg.
Copper	1.93 mg.
Potassium	1500 mg.
Inositol	150 mg.
Thiamin (B-1)	245 mcg.
Riboflavin (B-2)	240 mcg.

Niacin (B-3)	4 mcg.
Pyridoxine (B-6)	270 mcg.
Pantothenic acid	260 mcg.
Biotin	16 mcg.

What about other sweeteners? White sugar contains no nutrients and is pure carbohydrate. The best form of sugar, if you must use it, is Yellow D sugar. It is a rich brown sugar made from cane molasses and it contains natural vitamins and minerals. It is called a raw sugar. Turbinado sugar is also acceptable. Fructose—fruit sugar— is now also available.

Better than raw sugar as a sweetening, however, is natural unrefined, unclarified and unheated honey. If it is unprocessed and unrefined, it contains vitamins and minerals. Honey labeled as "pure, deluxe" and so clear that you read the label through it is robbed of its nutrients, so that it will look pretty. Reject it in favor of the cloudier, natural honey. That found in the comb is probably even richer, nutritionally, because it has not been tampered with in any way. In any case, go easy on *any* sweetener, which can perpetuate a "sweet tooth." Try to wean yourself from a craving for sweets by gradually using less and less.[7]

To produce molasses, sap from the sugar cane is collected. The first extraction, after boiling, is crystallized raw sugar (such as Yellow D). Usually it is later refined into pure white sugar thus being robbed of all nutrients. It encourages tooth decay, low blood sugar and a host of other ailments because it robs the body of B vitamins.

The second extraction produces a light molasses, richer in vitamins and minerals than raw sugar. Blackstrap, the third and last extraction, at the bottom of the barrel, so to speak, is the richest of all. Most of the nutrients have settled there. If you hear that blackstrap molasses includes straw, dirt and other extraneous material, pay no attention. It has served people well for centuries, and has improved health. It contains more calcium than milk, more iron than many eggs, more potassium than any food and is an excellent source of B vitamins. It contains no sugar at all. It can be added to yogurt, used for cooking. If it is taken straight, the mouth should be rinsed immediately, because any sticky substance encourages tooth decay. Blackstrap has been found to recolor hair in some cases, has prevented anemia (because of its high iron content) and has even been credited with stopping falling hair. Other acceptable natural sweeteners include honey (in small amounts), in liquid or crystallized form, and a rice/barley syrup.

LIVER

Liver has been considered one of the best "health foods" for many years. It contains vitamin B-12, and doctors and nutritionists advise eating it once or twice weekly. It provides protein, vitamins, minerals and energy, as proved by experiments with laboratory animals. Many doctors consider it a necessity for regaining or maintaining health. One physician says: "Adding liver to your diet invariably has resulted in a lasting improvement, often evident within a few days."

The reason liver is so effective is that it is a depot of all vitamins and minerals taken into the body. This is a plus factor, but there is a minus factor in our present-day polluted civilization. The liver is also a depot for poisons and pesticides which can lodge there in the fatty tissues. (Pesticides are always stored in fat.) For this reason many people are afraid to eat liver these days. Fortunately, there are several solutions to the problem. Organically raised meat does not come in contact with pesticide sprays or other chemical poisons. Therefore organic liver is safer. But some people do not like liver. In this case, desiccated liver, dried at low temperature to retain the nutrients, can be taken in powder or tablet form. One company derives its liver from animals raised in Argentina, where sprays are not used. Other companies now de-fat their desiccated liver which removes not only the fatty tissue but the pesticides and other poisons stored there. Liver from younger animals is said to be safer.

Liver has been given (in desiccated form) to athletes to provide stamina. It, too, has recolored some cases of prematurely gray hair. It is a powerhouse of nutrients and, in its safer forms, should be high on your list of high-power foods.

ANALYSIS OF LIVER

(in 100 grams or about 4 ounces fresh liver—an average slice)

Calcium	8 mg.
Phosphorus	486 mg.
Iron	7.8 mg.
	(hamburger contains only 2.8)

Vitamins:

A	53,500 I.U.
	(hamburger contains none)
B-1	.26 mg.
	(hamburger contains .08)
B-2	3.96 mg.
	(hamburger contains 1.19)
B-3 (niacin)	14.8 mg.

	(hamburger contains 4.8)
C	31 mg.
	(hamburger contains none)
B-12	35-50 mcg.
	(hamburger contains 2–5 mcg.)

From Heinz Nutritional Data, Fifth edition, published by Heinz Research Center.

SPROUTS

Many seeds and nuts are nutritionally rich. They contain vitamin E (the germ for regrowth upon planting) as well as protein, other vitamins and minerals. They are most nutritious when eaten raw, since cooking destroys much of their value. However, there is a way of using seeds that really hits the jackpot, nutritionally—sprouts from seeds. You can sprout them at home, or buy them already sprouted at the health store and some supermarkets. They can be germinated from any whole unhulled seeds or beans. The most popular are mung, soy, alfalfa and wheat. If you grow them yourself, do *not* buy those seeds coated with fungicides, mercury or other poisons. The coatings, usually vividly colored, may be *deadly*! These are usually found at seed stores. Those at the health stores are safe.

The Chinese, of course, have used bean sprouts for centuries. Sprouts can be added to salads, sandwiches, or dropped at the last minute into soups, casseroles or omelets, so that they will remain crisp and not be damaged by cooking at high heat.

Each person who sprouts seeds has his favorite method. I like mine because it is so simple and easy. Soak the seeds overnight. In the morning drain them. Place a white paper towel in a colander. Spread the seeds, one layer thick, on the towel. Cover with another paper towel. Hold the whole thing under the water tap and gently allow cold water to run over the towels, soaking them and the seeds. Drain again. Put the colander away in the corner of the kitchen counter and forget about it until the next morning. At this time, re-irrigate in the same way.

Dampen the seeds every morning. Within a few days they will develop little "tails" or sprouts. When these are about an inch long, remove the towels, wash the sprouts and refrigerate them.

A friend of mine lived next door to a physician. Both had children, and my friend always kept a bowl of sprouts on the table for the children and their friends to eat as snacks after school. They loved them. Later, the physician and his family moved away. After some time had passed he wrote: "As long as we lived next door to you, our children remained healthy. Since we have moved, they have been less healthy. The only way I can account for this change is that the sprouts must have contributed to their health.

"We are going to make them a habit in this family from now on," the doctor concluded.

There is no doubt that sprouts are nutritious; they contain a fantastic amount of vitamins B, C and E. When seeds sprout, the vitamin content increases, depending upon the vitamin, 10, 50, 100, 500 and 1,000 percent. They are one of the cheapest sources of natural (not synthetic) vitamins you can find.

Catharyn Elwood tells the full story of the increase of the vitamin content of sprouts.[8] I am going to quote one analysis to give you an idea of how sprouting seeds increases their value.

ANALYSIS OF B VITAMINS
IN SPROUTED OATS

Niacin	500% increase
Biotin	50% increase
Pantothenic acid	200% increase
Pyridoxine	500% increase
Folic acid	600% increase
Inositol	100% increase
Thiamin	10% increase
Riboflavin	1350% increase

We come to the end of this discussion of high-power foods. Don't let anyone kid you into thinking there are no such things as wonder foods.

REFERENCES

1. *Medical World News.* May 17, 1968.

2. Linda Clark. *Secrets of Health and Beauty.* Paperback edition. New York: Berkley-Jove, 1979.

3. The United States Department of Agriculture. *The Yearbook of Agriculture,* 1950–1951.

4. The United States Department of Agriculture. *The Yearbook of Agriculture,* 1959.

5. Evan V. Shute. *The Heart and Vitamin E.* Paperback edition. New Canaan, Conn.: Keats Publishing, 1977.

6. Beatrice Trum Hunter. *Yogurt, Kefir & Other Milk Cultures.* New Canaan, Conn.: Keats Publishing, 1973.

7. Linda Clark. *Stay Young Longer* (see chapter 7 on sugar). New York: Pyramid Books, 1968.

8. Catharyn Elwood. *Feel Like a Million.* New York: Pocket Books, Inc., 1965.

19
Protein,
the Real Staff of Life

Your body is made of protein. All parts of your body are dependent upon protein in some way for survival. Lack of protein weakens your muscle tone and makes you flabby. Without protein your facial muscles begin to droop and your skin begins to shrivel and wither. Adelle Davis said: "Since your body structure is largely protein, an undersupply can bring about age with depressing speed ... muscles lose tone, wrinkles appear, aging creeps in; and you, my dear, are going to pot."[1]

No living being survives without protein. The word *protein* was coined by a Dutch chemist in 1839 and means "of first importance." Protein is the stuff of life as you will soon see, but I prefer to call it the staff of life. Bread, formerly called the staff of life, no longer qualifies. But protein does. Hear this:

Hormones that regulate our bodies are proteins.

Our genes are protein.

The secretions of the thyroid gland, and the pituitary (the master gland) are proteins.

Insulin, the secretion of the pancreas, is a protein.

Antibodies, which protect you against infection, are proteins.

Enzymes, which perform a myriad of jobs in your body, are proteins.

The red coloring matter in your blood (hemoglobin) is a protein.

Your heart, liver, kidneys and eyes are made of protein.

Your hair and skin are about 98 percent protein.

Prolonged protein deficiency can cause: Anemia, kidney disease, liver disease, peptic ulcer, poor wound healing, lack of resistance to infection, irritability, fatigue, low blood pressure, nerve instability, low blood sugar (hypoglycemia), weakness, wasting, high cholesterol, poor circulation, constipation, mental retardation in children, poor vision and edema or water retention (reducers, please take note).

In other words, you need a continuous *daily* supply of sufficient protein in order to maintain your body at the top peak of efficiency. Protein cannot be stored in the body for long. When the supply is depleted, the body is forced to feed upon itself, causing tissue and muscle breakdown in all parts of it.

This information about protein and its effect upon the body is new. George K. Anderson, M.D., of the Council on Foods and Nutrition of the American Medical Association, stated in 1954 that the knowledge that protein is a preventive and curative food substance had developed only within the last few years. He stated that though there were noticeable effects from a temporary deficient intake of food proteins, a protein deficiency over a prolonged period of time could bring about the ailments I have just listed. There is no guarantee that inner changes are not taking place during a temporary deficiency. Many disturbances do not appear overnight. The damage is taking place behind the scenes and can eventually erupt as a time bomb.

How much protein should one eat daily? The general recommendation is 1 gram of protein for every 2.2 pounds of body weight. If you divide your weight by two, you will get the approximate amount of grams of protein you need daily.

However, the recommended amounts of protein vary in different countries. No one can quite agree, except that pregnant women as well as those breast-feeding their babies need more; people who have been ill need more (for repair purposes); and men need more than women do. The recommendation in this country is 65 grams of protein daily for men, and 55 for women. This recommendation, however, is considered low by other countries. In Sweden, hardworking laborers were found to need 189 grams daily; Russian laborers, 132; German soldiers, 145; Italian laborers, 115; French workmen, 135; and English workmen, 151. (The British Medical Association believes that a realistic allowance should be between 80 and 100 grams daily for the average person.)

Most people today are living on high carbohydrate diets which cause overweight, fatigue, irritability and vulnerability to illness. As we have already mentioned, if your diet is full of all the necessary minerals, you may need less protein. But in addition to a high man-made carbohydrate diet (which, except for fresh fruits, is usually lacking in minerals), most people are eating a low mineral diet, making sufficient protein a must for weight control, health and vitality. You know, no doubt, that athletes are required to eat a high protein diet, to provide stamina. *You* need stamina, too.

What kind of protein is best? Animal protein is similar to that of the human body, so nutritionists consider it preferable. Animal protein includes meat, fish, fowl, milk and eggs. These proteins are *complete* proteins, meaning that they contain *all* the essential protein factors, known as the amino acids. There are twenty-two of these amino acids; some are essential, some nonessential. The body MUST have all the essential amino acids in order to synthesize protein and maintain its protein balance. Animal feeding experiments have shown that the body needs all of the essential amino acids in *each* meal. If one or more of the essential or important amino acids is missing at one meal, it cannot be made up for by another meal even four hours later. As an example, gelatin, which you may take in water or juice, is an incomplete protein, and thus, if you take it alone, you are not getting all the amino acids your body needs at one time. If you were to combine it with bouillon (made from meat), you would have a complete protein. Soybeans, as well as brewer's yeast and wheat germ, are complete proteins. Most plant proteins are not complete. Here is a list of complete proteins and their equivalents in grams, showing how much you have to eat to get your daily quota of 80 grams per day, according to the British Medical Association. Frances Moore Lappé's books help here.[2]

COMPLETE PROTEINS

	Amount	Grams of Protein
Soybean flour, low fat	1 cup	60
Wheat germ	½ cup	24
Brewer's yeast, powdered	½ cup	50
Eggs	1	6

Milk, whole, skim or buttermilk 1 quart		32–35
Cottage cheese	½ cup	20
American or Swiss cheese	2 slices	10–12
Soybeans, cooked	½ cup	20
Meat, fish or fowl	¼ pound (approx. 1 serving)	15–22

What about vegetarians? Can't they be healthy without using animal protein? The answer is yes and no. Yes, if the vegetarian knows how to compute his amino acids; no, if he doesn't. If you depend upon protein foods other than animal proteins, you have to be a brain to make the grade. One vegetarian I know who remains healthy, vital and energetic, occasionally eats some fish and fowl and relies heavily on brewer's yeast to make up his daily protein quota. At night he takes a pad and pencil and figures out his number of grams as well as his amino acids for the day. If his gram count is low, he makes up the deficit before bedtime. It can be done, but it is hard work.

The best sources of vegetable proteins are legumes (certain peas and beans) seeds and sprouts, some grasses and some nuts. The soybean is the most complete protein of all vegetables. Brewer's yeast is an excellent high-protein, nonmeat food. It is cheaper than meat and can be grown within days or less, whereas it takes many months or more to grow animals for food. The greatest drawback of vegetable protein (even brewer's yeast, unless it is especially bred to contain it) is a complete lack of vitamin B-12. This is serious, and vegetarians have been found to have a lower amount of B-12 in their blood serum than nonvegetarians. A B-12 deficiency can sneak up on you and result in pernicious anemia. Adelle Davis warned vegetarians that they are subject to pernicious anemia unless they use milk and eggs in generous amounts. She said: "People who have followed a vegetarian diet without milk or eggs for five years or longer often develop sore mouths and tongues, menstrual disturbances, and a variety of nervous symptoms including a 'needles and pins' feeling in hands and feet, neuritis, pain and stiffness in the spine and difficulty in walking."[3]

Those who are lactovegetarians (meaning that they drink milk and eat eggs and other dairy products, but no meat, fish or fowl) have an excellent health record. Vegetarians who do not take these precautions often argue: "But I feel so good on beginning a vegetarian diet!" That word, "beginning," is the clue. The person is probably eating more fresh fruits and vegetables, which supply more minerals, and at first the protein shortage is not apparent. It may take months or even years for the explosion of that time bomb, but it does happen and I have seen it happen. On quick recall I can think of three people who have been vegetarians for several years. One woman is suffering from pain in the spine that continues day and night. Nothing has been found to give her permanent relief. Another woman, for many years on a vegetarian diet, developed heart trouble, kidney trouble and is constantly bloated with water, making her appear overweight, which she actually isn't. She finally made her choice to discontinue vegetarianism and is feeling better and looking better. The third person, a comparatively young man, has also been on a vegetarian diet for many years. He is suffering from excruciating pains in his hands and feet; his nerves are raw; he cannot sleep but a few hours; he is in constant torment. He, too, has turned against vegetarianism, but it is too late for repair to his nerve degeneration, a common aftermath of B-12 deficiency. Even if these vegetarians add B-12 at this late date, it may not be absorbed, since poor assimilation of both B-12 and protein is a direct result of a prolonged vegetarian diet.

But, you will say: "Our meat, fish and fowl are not fit to eat these days." You are right, not all of them are. Meat is treated with hormones. Chickens are, too, and grown as quickly as possible for the market. Fish (specially shellfish) are being contaminated with mercury and pesticides that have invaded the water. The solution here is to look for organic meat and poultry (available at most health stores) and get fish you know has come from *deep-sea levels*. Such food is harder to get and also more expensive than the run-of-the-mill supply at supermarkets. But maintaining good health these days costs money, though not nearly as much as drugs and hospitalization. Many a family has cut its drug and other health costs by returning to good organic food. This, too, presents a pitfall. Many suppliers are finding out that "organic" is a magic word and are claiming that food is organic when it is not. Health stores are the more trustworthy in this respect. If in doubt, ask for proof. (See Chapter 1.)

In the plant family, scientific reports show that proteins from wheat and wheat concentrates, plus soy flour, have satisfactory biological protein value but also have limited digestibility. Oat flour-soy flour mixtures were found to be almost completely compensated for in poor digestibility, at least as compared with milk, by the very high protein biological value.[4] Buckwheat protein was found closest to animal protein of all plant sources.[5] According to Beatrice Trum Hunter, soy flour is an allergen for many people; it can cause edema and flatulence (gas).

If you truly wish to learn how to compute amino

acids there is help for you. There is an excellent little book by Frances Moore Lappé that tells you how to do it.[6] Study the method and by following the rules, you can become a successful vegetarian, providing you also get B-12 in some way. This is crucial.

B-12 needs an "intrinsic factor" to make oral assimilation possible. This factor is now available by prescription only. There are a few brands of vitamin B-12 at health stores that include the B-12 absorption factor in another form.

Read your labels. The only other solution is to take B-12 injections, which guarantee its reaching your blood and cells by circumventing the digestive tract where it is unlikely to be picked up.

For you who are reducing, I call your attention to one other problem in following the plant combinations in order to establish a protein balance. Animal protein and dairy products are made almost entirely of protein. Grain cereals and legumes (beans and peas) are higher in carbohydrates. The animal-dairy products also contain some fat, which the body needs; the plants do not. You must make the decision whether to be firm and lean on an animal and/or dairy product diet, or risk overweight on a processed-carbohydrate-high vegetable protein diet.

In any event, this is still not the whole story for success in order to thrive on *any* kind of protein. You must first digest it. Many people complain that meat (or brewer's yeast) or something else—they are not sure what—does not agree with them. They may say either that they suffer from gas or that their food just sits there in their stomach and feels like a lump, or a rock or a stone. This may very possibly be due to a lack of hydrochloric acid. I have written this problem up fully in my book *Secrets of Health and Beauty*.[7] It tells how to find out if you have a lack of hydrochloric acid (usually known as HCl), what kind to use and how much to take. I will not repeat the information here except in summary.

HCl is a digestive acid secreted in normal stomachs. It digests protein, and the minerals calcium and iron. Without HCl, you can be in trouble. Many people decide, after watching TV commercials, that they have an overacid problem or heartburn, and take an antacid. Because the symptoms of too little acid are *exactly the same* as too much acid, it is the worst possible thing they can do. Dr. Hugh Tuckey, an expert on HCl, states that the only way to find out is to use the trial-and-error method, since few doctors understand this problem. He suggests taking an HCl tablet (he prefers HCl Betaine-plus-pepsin, from health stores) after a protein meal. If you find that lump feeling or the gas subsiding, you have solved your problem: a lack of HCl. If, on the other hand, you feel a burning sensation in your stomach, it may really be too much acid, a very rare occurrence, Dr. Tuckey says. If this happens, you simply drink a glass of water, which flushes away the extra HCl and the sensation should stop promptly.

What causes a lack of this natural digestant? Stress, anger, bickering at the table, worry before eating, as well as the hustle and bustle of our daily living. It used to be that only older people, as they became older, suffered from this form of indigestion (and didn't know what to do about it). Now, stress of any kind, as well as the lack of B vitamins or protein, can be a cause at any age. Even some babies lack HCl. When a few drops of the liquid form are added to their formulas, formerly puny infants begin to thrive.

Deficiencies of various vitamins and minerals can also cause a lack of HCl.

More and more people are becoming aware of the great value of HCl in helping them to digest protein *of any kind,* animal or vegetable or dairy. One nutritionally-oriented physician, who prescribes it routinely for most of his patients and witnesses the good effects, takes it himself, as I do, too. He says: "If I were marooned on a desert island and had only one nutrient to choose, I would take HCl." If you need it, and begin to use it, you will feel the same way.

REFERENCES

1. Adelle Davis. *Let's Eat Right to Keep Fit.* Paperback edition. New York: New American Library, 1970.

2. Frances Moore Lappé. *Diet for a Small Planet.* New York: Ballantine Books, 1975.

3. Adelle Davis. *Let's Get Well.* Paperback edition. New York: New American Library, 1972.

4. *American Journal of Clinical Nutrition.* September, 1972.

5. *Prevention.* November, 1972, p. 135.

6. Frances Moore Lappé, *op. cit.*

7. Linda Clark. *Secrets of Health and Beauty.* Paperback edition. Berkley-Jove, 1979.

See also:

Rudolph Ballentine. *Diet & Nutrition.* Honesdale, Pa.: Himalayan Institute, 1978.

20
You Can See
the Difference

Is THERE really a difference between natural and synthetic vitamins and minerals? Some supplement companies produce products from natural sources exclusively. Others make them from synthetics only. Still others combine both. Are all products the same in effect? What is the truth?

Most scientists claim that natural and synthetic vitamins and minerals are identical. Why do they believe this? How is a vitamin synthesized? Why is it synthesized?

The method of synthesis, generally speaking, is this: A single vitamin factor, called a crystalline substance, is separated from its natural source, such as rice polishings, brewer's yeast, liver, citrus fruits, etc. It then becomes an isolated factor. Once it is isolated, its molecular formation or pattern is determined; then it is duplicated in the chemical laboratory by assembling component parts from chemicals already available. Some of these chemicals are coal-tar products. The synthetic vitamins are then presumably identical to the natural crystalline vitamins which they imitate. They have the same molecular formations and the same chemical reactions, according to chemists who insist that no one can tell the difference.

Why are vitamins synthesized? Because synthetics are cheaper to produce than the natural.

However, though the isolated factor may appear identical, there is one undisputed difference between a natural and a synthetic product. Natural vitamins are derived or condensed from natural foods. In these natural foods many factors occur together: vitamins, minerals, amino acids and enzymes, which help the body utilize absorbable nutrients. Researchers are learning that *all of these factors work as a team*. When one is separated or torn away from the companions with which it grew, the natural balance is disturbed.

Nutrition research is finding that when these associated factors—known or unknown—are separated or removed, their utilization within the body is often disturbed. There are hundreds of examples already known, and more are being discovered as time passes. For example, it is already well known that vitamin D is needed for the assimilation of calcium. Calcium and phosphorus work as a team. Vitamin A is now reported to enhance the assimilation of vitamin E. Vitamin K has recently been found to protect against a deficiency of vitamin C. Usually these factors occur together in nature.

John J. Miller, Ph.D., a biochemist who has spent a lifetime studying these interrelationships, believes that man has not identified all the nutrients—nor the necessary interrelationships between the nutrients—let alone learned how to apply them to health. He says that man does not know all the elements which exist in plants and natural foods, nor how these nutrients are combined into a balance of vitamins, minerals, amino acids (protein factors) and enzymes.

Dr. Miller states, "We simply do not know enough . . . [to] ever be able to improve on Nature's plan of enzyme interrelationships."

Is this proof that natural vitamins are better?

The late Eugene Schiff explained it this way: "I believe it is wrong to say natural vitamins are better. In their crystalline or isolated form they may not be. The right way to say it is that natural vitamin *preparations* made from the whole foods or food concentrates are better to the extent that they contain other factors besides the individual vitamin. . . .

"If we want, for instance, one milligram of natural vitamin B-1 or thiamin, we do not put into a tablet one milligram of natural vitamin B-1, but 200 milligrams of yeast. The real difference in what the user gets in the other 199 milligrams present in the yeast, the associated factors which obviously cannot be present in one milligram of straight or synthetic B-1."

How can you tell whether a preparation is natural? Labels may give a clue. For example, to determine whether vitamin E is from synthetic or natural sources, the vitamin E can be examined in the laboratory by a chemical process. In natural vitamin E the molecules rotate light to the right, called dextro-rotatory or abbreviated as d. Synthetic E, examined by this same laboratory process, reveals equal portions of right and left molecules, designated by the letters dl. The average buyer cannot make this test himself, so he must search the labels, which unfortunately change from time to time. However, any vitamin E preparations marketed today are natural if they have the following labels*:

---

*Courtesy of J. R. Carlson Laboratories, Inc., Chicago, which specialize in natural vitamin E.

    d-alpha tocopherol
    d-alpha tocopheryl acetate
    d-alpha tocopheryl succinate
    mixed tocopherols

Synthetic vitamin E preparations which are marketed today will be labeled as follows:
    dl-alpha tocopherol
    dl-alpha tocopheryl acetate
    dl-alpha tocopheryl succinate [from Europe]

Buy other vitamins from a reputable firm specializing in natural vitamins.

Does this mean that you should avoid synthetic vitamins completely? Not necessarily. Studies show that certain fish cannot live in synthetic or artificial sea water, but when some natural sea water is added to the artificial, they can exist. Studies also show that certain isolated synthetic vitamins accomplish specific actions, i.e., nudging a sluggish or deficient cell or organ or tissue back into working order. However, many nutritional physicians feel that administration of these synthetic vitamins in massive amounts should be medically supervised. The reason: After the necessary stimulation has been achieved (nutritional physicians can determine this), the large amounts of synthetics become similar in action to drugs. Their continued administration is like whipping a tired horse. At that point, nutritional physicians believe, natural vitamin *preparations*, complete with *all* nutrients, known and unknown, should be used as maintenance therapy. They consider them safer in the long run. But there is another reason.

All due credit should go to the chemists who have isolated and synthesized vitamin factors. They have proved helpful in certain circumstances, as just described. But Rudolph Hauschka, D.Sc., has been at work for

decades on laboratory experiments which show the dis-
similarity between natural and synthetic vitamins and
the difference in their effect. He explains how we learned
about vitamins in the first place. In 1882 one group of
animals was fed synthetic milk, while another group
was given natural milk. The animals fed fresh milk grew
up to be lively; those on synthetic milk died. The
logical conclusion was that there must be "something"
in natural milk which had escaped chemical detection,
but was important to life. This hypothetical substance
was later (in 1912) called a "vitamin." This led to a tidal
wave of research and the discovery of many vitamins.
However, nutrition is in its infancy. We still have not
discovered all the factors in food. Twenty years ago
vitamin B-12 was thought to be the final discovery in
the B complex. Today we know there is a vitamin B-22,
and there are no doubt more to come.

An experiment in Dr. Hauschka's laboratory ascertained that single synthetic substances were indistin-
guishable from the natural, according to available tests,
but it was found that there was a difference in *effect*.
The doctor learned that synthetics of coal-tar origin are
effective *only in allopathic dosage* (i.e., usual drug
dosages), *but in homeopathic dilutions they are useless*.
He says, "Thus it is fair to say that a basic biological
difference exists between natural and synthetic products,
despite their chemical identity. Laboratory experiments
prove this."[1]

Now for a surprise. Other scientists have found a way
to distinguish a natural vitamin formula from a synthetic.
The sensitive crystallizations of natural nutrients *can be
photographed*. The results, called "chromatograms," look
a little like snowflakes but are in color. An analysis of
foods, or natural substances, by these chromatograms
will show a definite pattern, whereas the synthetics will

not have a pattern. The natural patterns can be translated into vitamin and mineral organizations. Those which have no pattern are considered by the researchers who discovered this process to be non-nutritious and valueless as foods.

Dr. Gerhard Schmidt of Switzerland, a follower of Rudolf Steiner, has long worked in this field. He has photographed chromatograms which reveal the differences between soils treated with chemical fertilizers and those treated with natural fertilizers. The difference, as proved by the chromatograms, is also visible in the foods grown on these soils (i.e., the chromatogram of an organically grown carrot differs from one grown as usual). Chromatograms also show the effect processing has on natural foods. For example, a chromatogram shows that strength is taken away from rice when it is "peeled" and polished. And flour which is stone-ground appears different from that produced by the commercial milling process which removes many natural factors.[2]

This is truly exciting news!

Actually, this method of photographing the crystalline structure in food elements is not new. About 1903, a Dr. Abbott in Australia was the first to experiment with the idea, using osmosis. Later, around 1926, the Doctors Kolisko, a man-and-wife M.D. team, improved upon the Abbott process, combining osmosis with metalized crystallization. They called this method "Capillary Dynamolytical Testing." These two doctors devoted their lives to this subject and made millions of experiments on natural foods. Their rare book, now out of print but soon to be reprinted, is called *Agriculture of Tomorrow*.

The late Dr. Ehrenfried Pfeiffer, of the Biochemical Research Laboratories in this country, considered by many chemists as the greatest biochemist of our time, was a student of the Koliskos and brought the dynamolytical testing method to this country from England. Dr. Pfeiffer also photographed many chromatograms in his laboratory.

He stated, "Various undulations and spike formations in a pattern enable researchers to recognize biological activity and intrinsic values not revealed in highly refined or synthetic preparations."

References

1. Rudolph Hauschka, D.Sc. *The Nature of Substance*. London: Vincent Stuart Ltd., 1966. (German text, 1950.)
2. Dr. G. Schmidt. *Beitrage*. No. 24, 1966, through No. 29, 1968; Dornach, Switzerland.

21
How to Feel Better Within Days

Less than a week ago, I woke up one morning feeling blah. There is no other adequate description of the way I felt; I just felt blah! I was dragging, my energy level was low, and I felt as if I had had it!

This morning I woke up feeling marvelous, on top of the world, with energy to spare and that good-to-be-alive feeling. I made this change within a single week, and all by myself. You can do the same thing.

It happens to us all, no matter how healthy. As a matter of fact, Dr. Bernard Jensen, who has treated thousands of patients by natural methods, says that he has never seen a completely healthy person.[1] On top of this, we eat, drink and breathe the wrong things, become tense (which interferes with smooth body function) and perhaps we get too little regular exercise. The result: our digestions slow down, our bodies become choked with poisons, we become tired and feel miserable. Dr. Jensen says, "A tired body cannot eliminate, absorb, digest, plan, love or concentrate properly."

So what to do? Filling up on drugs merely makes matters worse. Drugs, unless used for emergency life-saving purposes, merely mask symptoms but do not remove them. In fact, many poisons stored in the body may be caused by drugs. I recall reading many years ago that during a detoxification diet, or a colonic (I don't remember which), a natural doctor found the body of one of his patients ejecting drugs which had been taken over forty years previously!

Going to a hospital for a rest cure is no good, since the poor hospital diet, plus the drugs they insist upon giving people, only make matters worse. Happily, there is something exciting happening in England, where a fringe-medicine hospital has been planned. It will provide such unorthodox medical treatments as homeopathy, acupuncture, osteopathy, nature cures, and even faith healing. The hospital will have five sections. It will have an education center for *doctors* to learn nutrition and unorthodox medicine. It will have a surgical wing for necessary surgery only. It will have a maternity wing for natural childbirth, as well as for education of mothers both before and after pregnancy. It will have a medical wing for chronically ill people suffering from asthma, bronchitis, cancer, diabetes, heart conditions, and so forth, with curative treatments taught for home use afterwards. Finally, there will be a chapel and meditation center for people of all religions. Music and color therapy will also be available here.[2] Three cheers for England! The United States should have one in every city; they would be swamped.

A third possibility for people who merely need a tune-up (as I did) would be a spa where you are both pampered and treated by natural methods.[3] This is a lovely idea, but not practical for me. I cannot leave my work responsibilities, home, or garden, in these days of hard-to-find help and property vandalism. So, since a spa was not in the cards for me, I had to figure out my own plan. I did and it worked. Here is how.

To begin with, I work hard, long hours. Dr. Jensen tells us that a rested body is the one which gets well. Many times overwork is the cause of physical problems. Getting away from it all may help some, but if you are still tense, you are defeating yourself, he says. So he advises letting go, mentally *and* physically, and letting recuperation take place.[4]

This I did. I finished up the most demanding deadlines, put my desk in order, the cover on my typewriter and shut the door to my office. I decided I would take four days—four blissful days—of doing only what I felt like doing, nothing I was supposed to do. I love my home, which is located in a healthful climate, but which I seldom have time to notice. The air is good, but I seldom take time to breathe it. I realized that I had everything I needed right where I was, and also where I was the most comfortable. But even if I had lived in an apartment in a city, I could have done most of the same things. It isn't where you are, but what you are doing there, I decided, which is important.

I chose light reading instead of heavy educational literature. I got out some knitting, not because I like it, but because it is relaxing and gives my mind a rest. I was then ready for the next step: a detoxification diet. I bought all the necessary supplies and was ready to go. I didn't even tell anyone I was going to follow this four-day program. Otherwise, friends would have tried to talk me out of it (as they often do a would-be reducer) or might even call in alarm at regular intervals to see how I was. I merely told my family I was going to rest for a few days, to which they said, "Hurray!"

You may know by this time, from reading my various

books and articles, that I do not believe in complete fasting. I, and a growing number of therapists, consider fasting (with no foods and water only) extremely dangerous. We are not living in biblical days, but in a polluted world. Our bodies, scientists tell us, are loaded with pesticides and other poisons from food, water and air. If we start to fast on water these poisons are released too quickly into the bloodstream and can cause self-poisoning, and severe illness in many cases.

So I did it the safe way: with cleansing juices, and a little fruit now and then, to slow down the poison excretion and dilute the effect on the body. Since detoxification takes place through the intestines, the lungs, the kidneys, and the skin, I helped these processes by getting a little sun on my skin every day, breathing deeply outdoors and sleeping as long as possible, including a daily nap. I also took a long, warm tub soak, daily. You can exercise or walk, although I didn't.

The cleaning dietary program I used is one I have used before and swear by. The first time I heard of it was from an assistant to the originator of the program, Stanley A. Burroughs, who has since left this country (I wish I knew where he is, to thank him). The assistant wrote to tell me of a patient who was bedridden with all sorts of minor ailments and was promised that the Burroughs program would bring miracles as well as get the patient out of bed in ten days. It did. I didn't believe it until I tried it myself, and since then I have mentioned it to numerous other people, all of whom agree that they, too, end up feeling absolutely wonderful. This program, which Mr. Burroughs calls the Master Cleanser, is designed to:

- dissolve toxins and mucus throughout the body
- cleanse the kidneys and the digestive system
- purify glands and cells

- eliminate all unusable waste and hardened material in the joints and muscles
- relieve pressure and irritation in nerves, arteries and blood vessels
- build a healthy bloodstream

Mr. Burroughs also states that using this program three or four times a year will do wonders for less serious or mild conditions, or can be used more often for more serious conditions. He recommends, as an average, sticking to it for ten days. As you know by now, I used it for only four days. But the results were remarkable for me. Others will have to decide for themselves how long to continue. I believe there is no point in letting yourself get weak; in fact, I would be inclined to think that *great* weakness might be a warning to STOP, or to continue only under a doctor's supervision.

The Program
(as outlined by Mr. Burroughs)

Combine the juice of ½ lemon with two tablespoons of a certain type of sweetening, and add to an 8 ounce glass of hot water. The sweeteners are a *must*, according to Mr. Burroughs, to balance the lemon and achieve desired results. The only sweetenings allowed are any kind of unsulphured molasses: Grandma's, Barbados, Louisiana, or blackstrap. Some people who have trouble with these since they are slightly laxative (though usually a good thing in a cleansing program), use pure maple syrup with Mr. Burroughs' blessing. He does not condone honey for this program.

You are to drink this concoction, he says, from 6 to 12 times a day, whenever you feel hungry. *Be sure to use a straw.* Both lemon juice and molasses, if left on the teeth, can erode enamel. In any case, rinse your mouth with clear water after taking, just to be sure. Take no other food during the full time of the diet.

Most people use the mixture about six times daily. If you are not eliminating properly, Mr. Burroughs suggests a herb laxative tea, available at health food stores.

Mr. Burroughs assures us that there is no danger in this program; the only thing you can lose, he says, is mucus, waste and disease. He says healthy tissue is not affected. But he warns *not* to vary the amount of lemon juice per glass.

Now I must confess that I cheated. I had just read that watermelon is a marvelous diuretic, so I rewarded myself each afternoon with a small serving of watermelon. And since the repetition is boring, I took some brewer's yeast in water or broth at noontime or alternated the lemon-juice drinks with tomato juice or some fresh, natural vegetable juice. I also took plenty of vitamin C to speed neutralization of any poisons, even though Mr. Burroughs does not approve of supplements taken during this cleansing program. (Sorry about that, Mr. Burroughs.) After all, blackstrap, which was my choice of sweetening, is loaded with natural iron, calcium, potassium, and B vitamins. Lemon juice also contains vitamin C.

Now what do you do *after* you have decided to stop this program? Mr. Burroughs' suggestions are: eat, as often as you are hungry, a soup made of fresh vegetables, or using brown rice. He believes that you should continue to drink liquids freely for two days after coming off the diet and take no meat, eggs, fish, breads, pastries, etc. On the third day he believes normal eating can be resumed. Coming off the program is crucial!

Meanwhile, now is the time to improve your overall diet. There is no point in going back to the old junk which helped to get you into the condition you have just tried to correct. This diet is a marvelous opportunity to get rid of some of your addictions. Where other people may become addicted to sugar or alcohol, I am a pushover for all of the good natural breads available in California. This is an easy way to acquire a spare tire. I have lost a bread addiction whenever I have followed this diet, a great benefit for me.

Other good things have happened to me, too. Although you may look a little seamy when you first get off the diet, this will change, since you will be feeling so good you can't help but look better soon. I also lose weight on the diet (some of it returns, but less if I give up that old bogey-for-me, bread). Other little nagging things disappear. I won't enumerate them since yours may differ from mine. What does apply to everyone I have watched on this diet, is that they all report they feel like a million dollars and usually soon look the part, too.

What I never can understand is why I don't do this oftener. It is such a quick and rewarding program, even for prevention purposes, without waiting until you feel miserable. So help me, from now on, I am going to repeat it three times a year.

Meanwhile, here is a salute to Stanley A. Burroughs, wherever you are, for originating the Master Cleanser. It really works. Thank you.

References

1. Dr. Bernard Jensen. *World Keys to Health and Longevity*. Escondido, Cal.: Omni Publishers, 1975.
2. *Here's Health* (English magazine). May 1975.
3. Robert and Raye Yaller. *The Health Spas: World Guidebook to Health Spas, Mineral Baths and Nature Cure Centers*. Santa Barbara, Cal.: Woodbridge Press Publishing Co., 1975.
4. *World Keys to Health and Longevity*.

Epilogue

Nutrition, a young science, is never a fully completed, closed subject. The information you have just read comprises most of the knowledge known so far. Tomorrow, something new may be added. All of us who are interested in this new, wonderful and exciting subject after witnessing health improvement in ourselves or others, cannot stop here. We must, and want to keep up with the new findings as they occur. Because the story is not and probably never will be finished, as more is learned from the teacher Nature, more results will be forthcoming. We cannot afford to miss a trick. We should keep reading anything and everything we can get our hands on to keep abreast and up to date.

Reliable magazines such as *Let's Live, Prevention, Health Quarterly (Plus Two)* and *Your Good Health* report new information regularly. New books by reliable nutrition reporters also enrich our store of growing information. Even newspapers are becoming interested and reporting new discoveries in this field. Add any shred of new information as it comes to light to your collection. You will find it rewarding.

Remember always, that although everyone is governed by the same general rules, each person is different and may have unique variations on the same theme. For example, everyone needs vitamin E, but different people require different types or amounts. Find your own pattern through experimentation until you discover a program which works for you.

One physician who has changed from orthodox drug therapy to nutritional therapy is doing uncalculated good with his patients in an unexpected way. Let me give just one illustration. A mother of a pre-college daughter told me the following story:

"My daughter was under par most of the time. I finally took her to this nutritionally oriented physician who used no halfway measures. He did not allow some junk food and some good food; he demanded that all food put into the mouth be organic, natural, raw or undercooked, and supplemented with natural vitamins and minerals. He said there was no room for compromise in his program if one wanted to get well and stay well.

"In order to prepare this food for my daughter, I had to prepare it for myself and my husband, a retired executive army officer, because it was just too much trouble to cook differently for just one person. The type of food was different and the preparation was different than what I had been taught as I grew up. But this whole, complete nutritional, wholesome, natural and delicious food became a new way of life for us all. Not only my daughter, but my husband and I began to feel better. It did not come overnight but it came. None of us will ever turn back again.

"Today my daughter has graduated from college,

married and has a baby. She follows the new plan of eating in her new family. Her child reflects the good nutrition his mother had during pregnancy as well as the good nutrition he is receiving since his birth. His health is perfect. So here are two families who have learned and set up a new way of life through optimum nutrition.

'I am sure that all of the many other patients of this doctor have done likewise. If the whole world will follow suit, we will have, instead of the present sickly population now so evident, a vital, healthy population, which can face problems with exuberance and equanimity, resulting from good health. In other words, life will be worth living rather than something to be endured. I never believed it before, but now I know it to be true: we are truly what we eat."

SUGGESTED ADDITIONAL READING

Abrahamson, E. M. and Pezet, A. W. 1971. *Body, Mind and Sugar*. New York: Jove.

Adams, Ruth and Murray, Frank. 1975. *Body, Mind and the B Vitamins*. New York: Larchmont Books.

——1975. *Megavitamin Therapy*. New York: Larchmont Books.

Airola, Paavo. 1974. *How to Get Well*. Phoenix, Arizona: Health Plus.

Altschul, A. M. 1965. *Proteins, Their Chemistry and Politics*. New York: Basic Books.

Bailey, Herbert. 1968. *Vitamin E: Your Key to a Healthy Heart*. New York: Arc Books.

Bieler, Henry G. 1973. *Food Is Your Best Medicine*. New York: Random House.

Bircher-Benner, M. 1978. *Prevention of Incurable Disease*. New Canaan, Connecticut: Keats Publishing, Inc.

Blaine, Tom R. 1974. *Mental Health through Nutrition*. New York: Citadel Press.

——1979. *Nutrition and Your Heart*. New Canaan, Connecticut: Keats Publishing, Inc.

Bricklin, Mark. 1976. *The Practical Encyclopedia of Natural Healing*. Emmaus, Pennsylvania: Rodale Press, Inc.

Cheraskin, E. and Ringsdorf, W. M. Jr. 1973. *New Hope for Incurable Disease*. New York: Arco Publishing.

Cheraskin, E., Ringsdorf, W. M. and Brecher, A. 1976. *Psychodietetics*. New York: Bantam Books.

Cheraskin, E., Ringsdorf, W. M. and Clark, J. W. 1977. *Diet and Disease*. New Canaan, Connecticut: Keats Publishing, Inc.

Clark, Linda. 1972. *Be Slim and Healthy*. New Canaan, Connecticut: Keats Publishing, Inc.

——1972. *Get Well Naturally*. New York: Arco Publishing.

——1972. *Light on Your Health Problems*. New Canaan, Connecticut: Keats Publishing, Inc.

——1968. *Stay Young Longer*. New York: Pyramid Communications.

Cleave, T. L. 1975. *The Saccharine Disease*. New Canaan, Connecticut: Keats Publishing, Inc.

Davis, Adelle. 1970. *Let's Eat Right to Keep Fit*. New York: New American Library.

—— Paperback edition 1972. *Let's Get Well*. New York: New American Library.

Fredericks, Carlton. 1975. *Eating Right for You*. New York: Grosset & Dunlap.

—— 1980. *Eat Well, Get Well, Stay Well*. New York: Grosset & Dunlap.

Fredericks, Carlton and Goodman, Herman. 1976. *Low Blood Sugar and You*. New York: Constellation International.

Goodhart, Robert S. and Shils, Maurice E. 1973. *Modern*

Nutrition in Health and Disease, 5th ed. Philadelphia: Lea & Febiger.

Grant, Doris. 1974. *Recipe for Survival.* New Canaan, Connecticut: Keats Publishing, Inc.

Hills, Hilda Cherry. 1976. *Good Food, Gluten Free.* New Canaan, Connecticut: Keats Publishing, Inc.

—— 1980. *Good Food, Milk Free, Grain Free.* New Canaan, Connecticut: Keats Publishing, Inc.

Hoffer, Abram and Osmond, Humphry. 1966. *How to Live with Schizophrenia.* New York: University Books.

Hoffer, Abram and Walker, Morton. 1980. *Nutrients to Age Without Senility.* New Canaan, Connecticut: Keats Publishing, Inc.

——1978. *Orthomolecular Nutrition.* New Canaan, Connecticut: Keats Publishing, Inc.

Hunter, Beatrice Trum. 1973. *The Natural Foods Primer.* New York: Simon and Schuster.

——Revised edition, 1980. *Additives Book.* New Canaan, Connecticut: Keats Publishing, Inc.

Jacobson, Michael F. 1972. *Eater's Digest.* Garden City, New York: Doubleday Anchor.

Kirban, Salem. 1979. *The Getting Back to Nature Diet.* New Canaan, Connecticut: Keats Publishing, Inc.

Kirschmann, John D., Nutrition Search, Inc. 1975. *Nutrition Almanac.* New York: McGraw-Hill.

Kugler, Hans J. 1977. *Dr. Kugler's Seven Keys to a Longer Life.* New York: Fawcett.

Lappé, Frances M. 1975. *Diet for a Small Planet.* New York: Ballantine Books.

Larson, Gena. 1972. *Better Food for Better Babies.* New Canaan, Connecticut: Keats Publishing, Inc.

McGee, Charles T. 1981. *How to Survive Modern Technology.* New Canaan, Connecticut: Keats Publishing, Inc.

Mervyn, Len. 1981. *Minerals and Your Health*. New Canaan, Connecticut: Keats Publishing, Inc.

Moyer, William C. 1971. *Buying Guide for Fresh Fruits Vegetables and Nuts*, 4th ed. Fullerton, California: Blue Goose.

Newbold, H. L. 1975. *Mega-Nutrients for Your Nerves*. New York: Berkeley.

Null, Gary and Null, Steve. 1973. *The Complete Handbook of Nutrition*. New York: Dell.

Page, Melvin E. and Abrams, H. L. 1972. *Your Body Is Your Best Doctor*. New Canaan, Connecticut: Keats Publishing, Inc.

Passwater, Richard A. 1976. *Supernutrition*. New York: Pocket Books.

Pauling, Linus. 1971. *Vitamin C and the Common Cold*. New York: Bantam.

Pfeiffer, Carl C. 1975. *Mental and Elemental Nutrients*. New Canaan, Connecticut: Keats Publishing, Inc.

Philpott, William H. and Kalita, Dwight K. 1980. *Brain Allergies: The Psycho-Nutrient Connection*. New Canaan, Connecticut: Keats Publishing, Inc.

Pinckney, Edward and Pinckney, Cathy. 1973. *The Cholesterol Controversy*. Los Angeles, California: Sherbourne Press.

Rodale, J. I. 1975. *The Complete Book of Vitamins*. Emmaus, Pennsylvania: Rodale Press.

——1976. *The Complete Book of Minerals for Health*. Emmaus, Pennsylvania: Rodale Press.

Rosenberg, Harold and Feldzaman, A. N. 1975. *The Doctor's Book of Vitamin Therapy*. New York: Berkeley.

Schroeder, Henry A. 1978. *The Poisons Around Us*. New Canaan, Connecticut: Keats Publishing, Inc.

—— 1971. *Pollution, Profits and Progress*. Brattleboro, Vermont: Stephen Greene Press.

Shute, Evan V. Paperback edition 1977. *The Heart and Vitamin E.* New Canaan, Connecticut: Keats Publishing, Inc.

Shute, Wilfrid E. 1978. *The Complete Vitamin E Book.* New Canaan, Connecticut: Keats Publishing, Inc.

Stone, Irwin. 1970. *The Healing Factor: Vitamin C Against Disease.* New York: Grosset & Dunlap.

Taylor, Renée. 1978. *Hunza Health Secrets.* New Canaan, Connecticut: Keats Publishing, Inc.

Thurston, Emory W. 1979. *Parents' Guide to Better Nutrition.* New Canaan, Connecticut: Keats Publishing, Inc.

Wade, Carlson. 1975. *Hypertension and·Your Diet.* New Canaan, Connecticut: Keats Publishing, Inc.

—— 1980. *Carlson Wade's Lecithin Book.* New Canaan, Connecticut: Keats Publishing, Inc.

Walker, Morton. 1979. *Total Health.* New York: Everest House.

——1980. *How Not to Have a Heart Attack.* New York: Franklin Watts, Inc.

——1980. *Chelation Therapy: How to Prevent or Reverse Hardening of the Arteries.* Seal Beach, California: '76 Press.

Williams, Roger J. 1973. *Nutrition Against Disease.* New York: Bantam.

Winter, Ruth. 1972. *Beware of the Food You Eat,* rev. ed. New York: New American Library.

Yudkin, John. 1972. *Sweet and Dangerous.* New York: Bantam.

INDEX

MEASUREMENT CONVERSION CHART

Water-soluble vitamins (the B and C vitamins) are measured in milligrams, occasionally (as in B-12) in micrograms.

One *gram* equals 1,000 milligrams, or one million micrograms

One *milligram* (mg) is 1/1000 of a gram (g)

One *microgram* is one millionth of a gram. A microgram is usually abbreviated as mcg, with one exception. A new British measurement is just beginning to be substituted as μg, which is the Greek equivalent of a microgram.

Fat-soluble vitamins (A, E, D, K) are measured in International Units (I.U.) except for one factor of vitamin A in micrograms expressed in μg.

WEIGHT OF DRIED FOODS (includes flour, rice, seeds, nuts)

One *pound* of dry food equals 16 ounces or 500 grams

One-half pound of dry food equals 250 grams

One *ounce* of dry food equals approximately 30 grams

Two pounds equal 32 ounces or one kilogram, which is 2.2046 pounds.

VOLUME—FLUID MEASUREMENTS (METRIC)

One *liter* equals 32 fluid ounces, or two pints, or four cups, or 1.057 quarts

One *gallon* equals four quarts or slightly less than four liters

One *tablespoon* equals three teaspoons, or 15 milliliters (ml)

One *milliliter* equals ⅕ teaspoon

One *teaspoon* equals ⅓ tablespoon, or 60 drops, or five milliliters

One *fluid ounce* equals two tablespoons or 30 milliliters

One *cup* equals 16 tablespoons, or eight fluid ounces, or ½ pint, or 250 milliliters

One *pint* equals 16 fluid ounces, or two cups, or 500 milliliters

One *quart* equals 32 fluid ounces, or two pints, four cups, or slightly less than one liter

(Measurements adapted from American National Standards Institute and Rodale Press. Amounts are approximate for convenience in using.)